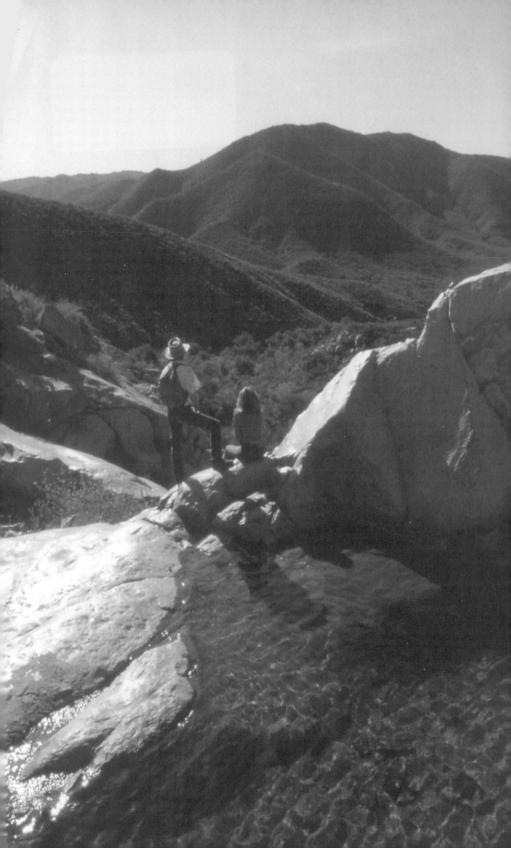

Afoot & Afield

Orange County
A comprehensive hiking guide

Jerry Schad

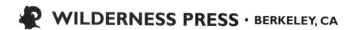 **WILDERNESS PRESS** · BERKELEY, CA

Afoot & Afield Orange County

1st EDITION 1988
2nd EDITION November 1996
3rd EDITION March 2006

Copyright © 1988, 1996, 2006 by Jerry Schad

Front cover photo copyright © 2006 by Jerry Schad
Interior photos, except where noted, by Jerry Schad
Maps: Jerry Schad
Cover design: Andreas Schuller / Larry B. Van Dyke
Book design and layout: Andreas Schuller / Larry B. Van Dyke
Book editor: Jessica Benner

ISBN-13 978-0-89997-397-5
ISBN-10 0-89997-397-3
UPC 7-19609-97397-3

Manufactured in the United States of America

Published by: **Wilderness Press**
1200 5th Street
Berkeley, CA 94710
(800) 443-7227; FAX (510) 558-1696
info@wildernesspress.com
www.wildernesspress.com
Visit our website for a complete listing of our books and for ordering information.

Cover photo: Santiago Oaks Regional Park
Frontispiece: Top of Tenaja Falls, San Mateo Canyon Wilderness

SAFETY NOTICE: Although Wilderness Press and the author have made every attempt to ensure that the information in this book is accurate at press time, they are not responsible for any loss, damage, injury, or inconvenience that may occur to anyone while using this book. You are responsible for your own safety and health while in the wilderness. The fact that a trail is described in this book does not mean that it will be safe for you. Be aware that trail conditions can change from day to day. Always check local conditions and know your own limitations.

Acknowledgments

Many people have offered their time, talents, and knowledge during the various phases of producing the first edition of this book. I would like to thank Ralph Davis, Beth Davis, Mike Fry, Janet Leavitt, Camille Armstrong, Don Nelson, Genie Rope, René Schad, Walton Scott, Bert Ton, Gene Troxell, John Welch, and Howie Wier for sharing adventures with me on the trail, and for helping with transportation. Several people associated with local parks and preserves and Cleveland National Forest have been of assistance too, among them Bill Bretz, Bruce Buchman, Lee Edwards, Ernie Martinson, Jim Snow, and Jon Wright. Ilse Byrnes provided information about Orange County's regional riding-and-hiking trail system. Tom Winnett of Wilderness Press, in his characteristic meticulous way, superbly edited the text.

Since the first edition of this book debuted in 1988, I've had the pleasure of re-hiking many familiar routes and exploring more than 30 new ones. As a result, there are 87 hiking trips in this current, third edition. For assistance or companionship in these endeavors, I wish to thank Bob Birkland, Lee Di Gregorio, Marian Mongar, Sky York, Susan Zahn, M.A. Durrin, Barbara Norton, John Strauch, Barbara Amato (whose likeness appears in this edition's cover photograph), DeNeice Kenehan, Rob Smith, Carl Johnson, Tom Chester, Steve Johnson, John Gustafson, Dan English, Debra Clarke, and Jim Campbell. Special appreciation is due to Juergen Schrenk, Dave Chamberlin, and Betsy Chamberlin, whose notes and accounts of recent hikes throughout Orange County were shared in detail with me.

I wish to thank Roslyn Bullas, who kept this revised, third edition moving through production; Jessica Benner, who edited the text; and Larry Van Dyke and Andreas Schuller, who synthesized the book's textual and graphic elements into a spacious and coherent whole.

Jerry Schad
La Mesa, California
January 2006

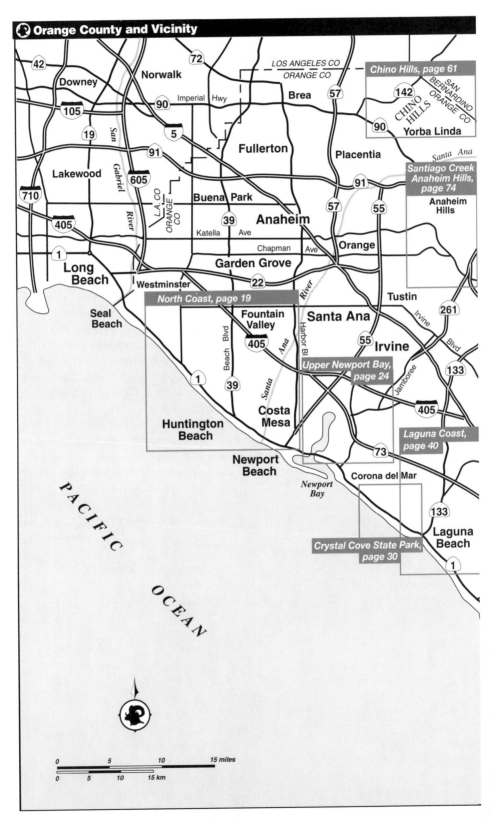

42
Downey
105
19
Lakewood
710
405
1
Long Beach
Seal Beach

Norwalk
72
Imperial Hwy
90
5
91
605
San
Gabriel
River
L.A. CO
ORANGE CO
Buena Park
39
Katella Ave
Westminster

Brea
57
Fullerton

Placentia

91
57   55

Anaheim
Chapman   Ave
Garden Grove
22

142
SAN BERNARDINO
ORANGE CO
CHINO HILLS
90
Yorba Linda

Santa Ana

Anaheim Hills

Orange

Tustin

Fountain Valley
405
Beach Blvd
39
1
Huntington Beach

Newport Beach

Santa Ana
55   Irvine

Harbor Bl
Santa Ana River

Costa Mesa

Newport Bay

Irvine Blvd
261
133
Jamboree
405

73
Corona del Mar

133
Laguna Beach
1

PACIFIC   OCEAN

LOS ANGELES CO
ORANGE CO

0   5   10   15 miles
0   5   10   15 km

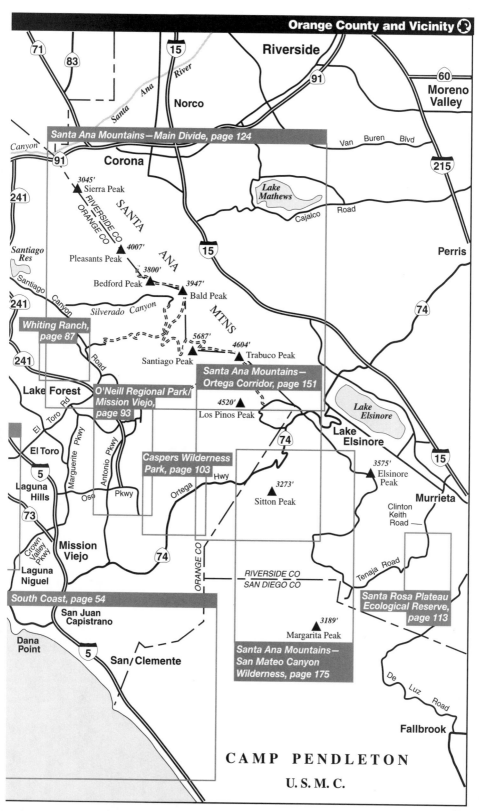

71

83

15

Riverside

71

River

60

91

Norco

Moreno Valley

215

Canyon

91

Corona

Van Buren Blvd

241

3045'
▲ Sierra Peak

Lake Mathews

RIVERSIDE CO
ORANGE CO

SANTA

Cajalco Road

Perris

Santiago Res

4007'
▲
Pleasants Peak

ANA

15

241

3800'
▲
Bedford Peak

3947'
▲
Bald Peak

MTNS

74

Santiago

Canyon

Silverado Canyon

241

5687'
▲
Santiago Peak

4604'
▲ Trabuco Peak

Road

Lake Forest

Toro

El

Lake Elsinore

Toro Rd

4520'
▲
Los Pinos Peak

El Toro

Marguerite Pkwy

Antonio Pkwy

Lake Elsinore

5

Laguna Hills

Oso

Pkwy

74

3575'
▲ Elsinore Peak

Murrieta

73

Hwy

3273'
▲
Sitton Peak

Clinton Keith Road

Crown Valley Pkwy

Mission Viejo

Ortega

ORANGE CO

Laguna Niguel

74

RIVERSIDE CO
SAN DIEGO CO

Tenaja Road

San Juan Capistrano

Dana Point

5

3189'
▲
Margarita Peak

5

San/Clemente

De Luz Road

Fallbrook

CAMP PENDLETON

U. S. M. C.

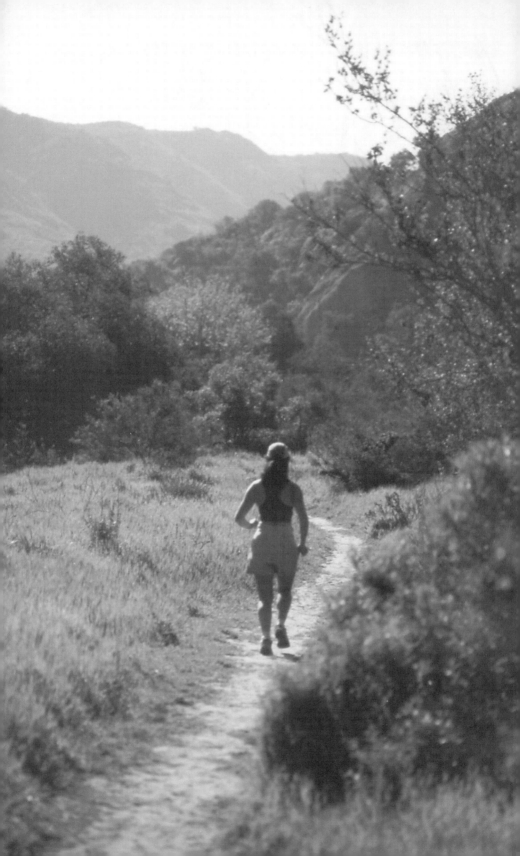

Contents

At the mouth of Laurel Canyon

Preface

Hidden within or just beyond Orange County's urban sprawl lies more opportunity for the appreciation of the natural world than most county residents would ever imagine. Barely a few hundred yards from busy highways and shimmering glass high-rises, shorebirds haunt protected estuaries and marshes. Along the southern coast, ocean swells roll in and spend themselves against lonely sands and jagged cliffs. Over the foothill country hawks and eagles cruise in search of a furry meal. And deep within the corrugated fastness of the Santa Ana Mountains mountain lions, deer, and coyotes roam cool, dark canyon bottoms and sun-warmed, chaparral-covered slopes.

Surrounding Orange County's densely populated coastal plain are parks, preserves, designated open spaces, and public lands totaling approximately 200,000 acres. Within this domain, intriguing pathways introduce explorers to natural landscapes ranging from the intertidal zone to oak and coniferous woodlands. Orange County boasts either within or abutting its rather compact border eight state parks and beaches, 19 regional (county) parks and wilderness areas, more than 130,000 acres of national forest, and more than 500 miles of trails and roads for hiking.

My goal in writing this guide was to bring into sharp focus virtually every walk worth taking on still-wild public lands conveniently accessible to the average Orange Countian. The hikes range in difficulty from short strolls through selected urban parks and preserves to canyon treks in the Santa Ana Mountains that would challenge any adventurer.

Because of Orange County's rather small area (782 square miles) but larger sphere of influence, a number of hikes in this book lie either partly or wholly outside the county boundaries. These are found in the following areas: Chino Hills State Park, extending into San Bernardino and Riverside counties; Santa Rosa Plateau Ecological Reserve in southwestern Riverside County; San Onofre State Beach in northern San Diego County; and the entire Trabuco Ranger District of Cleveland National Forest, spilling into Riverside and San Diego counties. (Two other units of the Cleveland Forest, the Palomar and Descanso districts, extend farther east and south across Riverside and San Diego counties. Those units, along with other public lands in San Diego County, are treated in my book *Afoot and Afield in San Diego County*. For those interested in hikes in and around Los Angeles, a third volume in the "Afoot and Afield" series is available: *Afoot and Afield in Los Angeles County*.)

Every trip in this book was hiked by me at least once at one time or another. Roads and trails can and do change, however. Publicly accessible open-space acreage is increasing, and new trails are being constructed and opened for public use. In the national forest, the greater demand for recreational use is leading to new regulations and new use patterns. I will continue to insert fresh updates in future printings of this edition, and a fourth edition will undoubtedly appear in the future. You can keep me apprised of recent developments and/or changes by writing me in care of Wilderness Press, 1200 Fifth Street, Berkeley, CA 94710, or e-mailing comments directed to me at mail@wildernesspress.com. I will appreciate your comments.

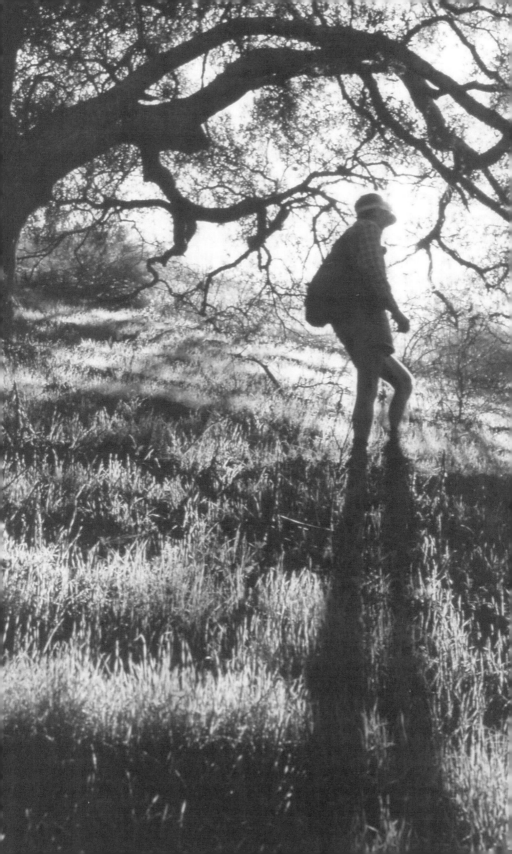

Introducing Orange County

From the look-alike cities in the north to the newer, planned communities of the south, Orange County seems little distinguished from its colossal neighbor and economic parent, Los Angeles. But a deeper identity, rooted in geography, transcends the urban sprawl. Orange Countians are reminded of their uniqueness not so much by the human architecture of city and suburb, but rather by the blue Pacific, the green and tawny coastal hills, and the purple wall of the Santa Ana Mountains.

Out on the coastline and up along the foothills and mountains, you may discover for yourself Orange County's place in the natural world. An hour or less of driving and less than two hours' walk will take you from the frenetic city to any of several interesting natural environments, ranging from tidepools to fern-bedecked canyon streams to mountain peaks affording views stretching a hundred miles. You'll discover fascinating rock formations, rich and varied plant life, a healthy population of native animals, and a sense of peace and tranquility.

In the next few pages of this book, we'll briefly introduce you to the "other" Orange County: its climate, geology, flora, and fauna. Following that, you'll find some notes about safety and courtesy on the trail, and some tips on how to get the most out of this book. After perusing that material, you can dig into the heart of this book—descriptions of 87 hiking routes from the coast to the Santa Ana Mountains. Happy reading and happy hiking!

Land of Gentle Climates

A succinct summary of Orange County's climate might take the form of just two phrases: "warm and sunny," and "winter-wet, summer-dry." But some variation in climate exists across the county's width from coast to mountain crests. Without resorting to technical classification schemes, let's divide the county into just two climate zones: The coastal zone, extending inland 10–15 miles across the coastal plain and low coastal foothills, is largely under the moderating influence of the Pacific Ocean. This climate is characterized by mild temperatures that are relatively unvarying, both daily and seasonally. Average Fahrenheit temperatures range from the 60s/40s (daily highs/lows) in winter, to 70s/60s in summer. Rainfall averages about 15 inches annually. Overall this climate closely matches the classic "Mediterranean climate" associated with coastal areas along the Mediterranean Sea.

The inland zone, consisting of the Santa Ana Mountains and foothills, experiences somewhat more extreme daily and seasonal temperatures, because it is less influenced by onshore flows of marine air. The higher summits of the Santa Ana Mountains, for example, have average temperatures in the 50s/20s in winter, and the 80s/50s in summer. Precipitation averages about 30 inches annually in the higher Santa Anas, which is just enough to support natural pockets of coniferous and broadleaf trees such as pines, oaks, and maples. Almost every year, some fraction of the precipitation arrives in the form of snow, which briefly blankets the mountain slopes down to an elevation of about 3000 feet.

Despite its reputation for gentle climate, Orange County is occasionally subject to hot, dry winds called "Santa Ana

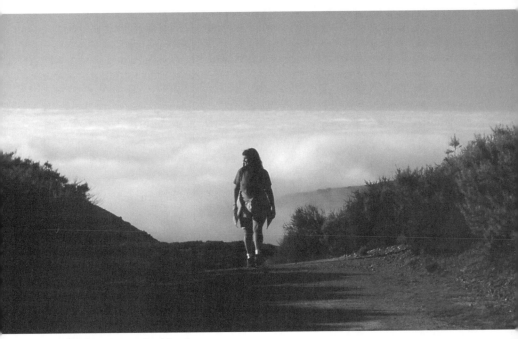

Cloud walking, Laguna Bowl Road

winds" (after Santa Ana Canyon, just north of the Santa Ana Mountains). These winds occur when an air mass moves southwest from a high-pressure area over the interior U.S. out toward Southern California. As the air flows downward toward the coast, it compresses and becomes warm and dry. Low passes in the mountains, or river valleys that act as wind gaps (such as Santa Ana Canyon), funnel these desertlike winds toward the coast. During stronger Santa Anas, common in late summer and fall, Orange County basks under warm, blue skies swept clear of every trace of pollution (except possibly smoke from wildfires). Temperatures along the coast can then reach record high levels; the city of Orange, for example, once recorded a temperature of 119 degrees during a Santa Ana.

Rainfall in Orange County is as erratic as it is slight. On the coastal plain, the annual precipitation has ranged from just 4 inches to a record of 32 inches. Up to 5 inches have fallen on the coastal plain in a single day, and in the Santa Ana Mountains one storm dumped 9 inches in a single night.

By and large, Orange County's balmy, dry climate is remarkably well suited to year-round outdoor activity. Nevertheless, high temperatures, scarcity of water, and occasionally smoggy air during summer and early fall make that particular period less desirable for hiking in the inland foothills and mountains. During the other seven or eight months of the year, the weather is often ideal.

Reading the Rocks

Of California's many geomorphic (natural) provinces, Orange County claims parts of just two: the Los Angeles Basin and the Peninsular Ranges. The bulk of the county's urbanized area lies in the Los Angeles Basin, while the mostly undeveloped Santa Ana Mountains and the semi-developed San Joaquin Hills belong to the Peninsular Ranges province.

The Los Angeles Basin province extends from the base of the San Gabriel and Santa Monica mountains (part of the Transverse Ranges province) on the north to the base of the Santa Ana Mountains and the San Joaquin Hills on the south. In a geologic context it can be pictured as a huge, deeply folded basin filled to a depth of up to 7 miles by some volcanic material and land-laid sediments, but mostly by sediments of marine origin—sand and mud deposited on the ocean bottom from 80 million years ago to as recently as 1 million years ago.

The Los Angeles Basin area has experienced uplift during the past 1–2 million years, and as this took place the surface of the basin accumulated a layer of terrestrial sediment shed from the surrounding hills and mountains. The basin, in fact, would be still be filling up with sediment today were it not for the flood-control dams and channeled riverbeds that have largely replaced the original meandering Santa Ana, San Gabriel and Los Angeles rivers.

Hikers following this guidebook will discover many interesting and sometimes colorful exposures of marine sedimentary rocks in places like the Chino Hills, the San Joaquin Hills, and the foothills of the Santa Ana Mountains. These sediments, uplifted by a variety of geologic processes, are continuations of the formations that lie deep underground in the center of the Los Angeles Basin.

The marine sediments you will see—sandstone, siltstone, shale, and conglomerate—tend to be rather soft and easily eroded. Along the south coast, where the San Joaquin Hills meet the sea, several wave-cut "marine terraces" are identifiable on the coastal headlands. They exhibit a record of changing sea levels and gradual uplift over the past one or two million years. In many places the terraces themselves are deeply cut by drainage channels—the coastal canyons —which themselves are quite recent features.

The Santa Ana Mountains, along with the San Jacinto Mountains, lie at the northwest tip of the extensive Peninsular Ranges province, stretching south toward the tip of Baja California (the province, in fact, derives its name from Baja's peninsular shape). Each range in this province possesses a core of granitic (granitelike) rock, overlain in many places by a veneer of older metamorphic rocks. Many of the Peninsular ranges, including the Santa Anas, are raised and tilted fault blocks, typically with steep east escarpments and more gradually inclined western slopes.

As you travel through the Santa Ana Mountains (and their distinctly named subdivisions, the Elsinore and the Santa Margarita mountains), you'll begin to piece together their geologic history. Starting at, say, Caspers Wilderness Park in the foothills and moving up toward the crest of the Santa Anas, you first pass among light-colored marine sedimentary rock formations that were pushed up and tilted by the rise of the mountains to the east. Next comes metamorphic rock of two basic kinds—metasedimentary and metavolcanic. These brown- or gray-colored rocks, roughly 200–150 million years old, are metamorphosed (changed by heat and pressure) forms of marine sedimentary and volcanic rock that were plastered against the core of the North American continent some tens of millions of years ago. These rocks were riding on one or more of the earth's tectonic "plates" which were colliding with and being "subducted" (forced under) the western edge of the continent.

Near the crest of the Santa Ana Mountains you find light-colored granitic rocks. Here's the reason: About 100 million years ago, when the subduction process was in full swing, much of the material on the edge of the plate being subducted was melting underground and accumulating in the form of vast pools of magma. Because this magma was less dense than the surrounding materials, it began rising toward the surface. Some escaped through volcanoes, but most of it remained underground long enough to slowly cool and crystallize, forming coarse-grained "plutonic" (generally granitic) rocks. Erosion then nibbled away at the overlying metamorphic rocks, finally exposing—typically in high places—the granitic rocks.

In the southern Santa Anas and throughout most of California's share of the Peninsular Ranges, this granitic rock is now well exposed. In the northern Santa Anas, however, its distribution is less extensive. The highest peaks in the range, Santiago and Modjeska peaks (together called Old Saddleback), are still covered by the older, overlying metamorphic rocks.

The granitic rocks are still rising today, more than offsetting the leveling effects of erosion. Thus, although the rocks of the Santa Ana Mountains range between old and ancient, the origin of the range itself as a structural unit is quite recent.

Of more than casual interest to Orange Countians is the fact that for at least the past 10 million years, the Peninsular Ranges province (along with the present Los Angeles Basin and a wedge of coastal central California) has been drifting northwest relative to the rest of the North American continent. In a global view, this motion is seen as a lateral sliding (or rather a repeated lurching) at the interface between the largely oceanic Pacific Plate and the largely continental North American Plate. The average rate of movement today is about 2 inches per year—enough, if it continues, to put Orange County abreast of San Francisco 12 million years from now.

The famous San Andreas Fault (which passes about 40 miles northeast of Orange County) is the principal division between the two plates. But earth movement can also take place along "splinter" faults south and west of the San Andreas. One such splinter fault, the Elsinore Fault, passes along the eastern base of the Santa Ana Mountains. Horizontal and vertical movements along this fault over the past 5 million years have shifted the Santa Ana Mountains northwest relative to the adjacent landforms to the east, and have raised and tilted the whole mountain block into the characteristic west-sloping orientation. Sudden earth movements along any of these faults have been and will again be responsible for most of Southern California's devastating earthquakes.

The geologic history of Orange County is a fascinating one, and the diversity of landforms and rocks in Orange County and the Santa Ana Mountains is enough to pique the curiosity of most any amateur geologist. Refer to Appendix 3 for sources of more information.

Native Gardens

About 800 different kinds of wild flowering plants are found within Orange County's 782 square miles, a remarkably large number when one considers its diminutive size among California counties.

Southern oak woodland, San Mateo Canyon Wilderness

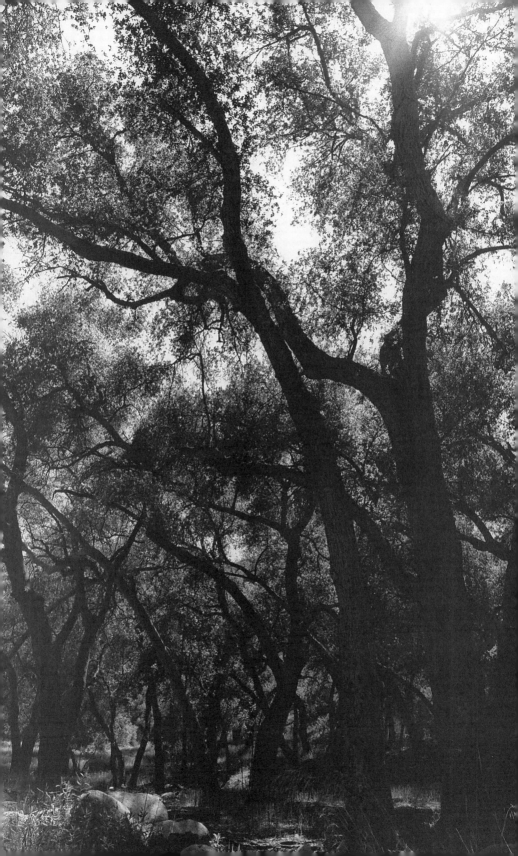

There are two reasons for this abundance of plant species. One reason has to do with physical factors: topography, geology, soils, and climate. Countywide, the diversity of physical factors and the complex interrelationships among these factors have led to the existence of many kinds of biological habitats.

The second reason is Orange County's location between two groups of flora: a southern, drought-tolerant group, most clearly represented by various forms of cacti; and a northern group, represented by moisture-loving plants typical of California's northern and central Coast Ranges. As the climate changed, varying from cool and wet to warm and dry over the past million years or so, species from one group and then the other invaded the county. Once established, many of these species persisted in protected niches even as the climate turned unfavorable for them. Some survived unchanged; others evolved into unique forms. Some are present only in very specific habitats.

The bulk of Orange County's undeveloped land can be grouped into three general classes, which botanists often call plant communities or plant associations. In a broader sense, these are biological communities, because they include animals as well as plants. These plant communities are briefly described below.

The *sage-scrub* (or coastal sage-scrub) community lies mostly below 2000 feet elevation, and extends east from the coastline to the foothills and lower spurs of the Santa Ana Mountains. The dominant species are small shrubs, typically California sagebrush, black sage, white sage, and wild buckwheat. Two larger shrubs often present are laurel sumac and lemonade berry, which like poison oak are members of the sumac family. Interspersed among the somewhat loosely distributed shrubs is a variety of grasses and wildflowers, green and colorful during the rainy season, but dry and withered during the summer and early fall drought.

The *chaparral* community is commonly found above 2000 feet elevation in the Santa Ana Mountains, where it cloaks the slopes like a thick-pile carpet. The dominant plants are chamise, scrub oak, manzanita, mountain mahogany, toyon, and various forms of ceanothus ("wild lilac"). These are tough, intricately branched shrubs with deep root systems that ensure survival during the long, hot summers. Chaparral is sometimes referred to as an "elfin forest" and that's a literal description of a mature stand. Without the benefit of a trail, travel through mature chaparral, which is typically 10–15 feet high, is almost impossible. Sage-scrub and chaparral vegetation tend to intermix readily throughout the Santa Anas, the chaparral preferring shadier, north-facing slopes, and the sage-scrub preferring hot, dry, south-facing slopes.

The *southern oak woodland* community is found in scattered locations throughout the county, from the bigger coastal canyons in the San Joaquin Hills to moist flats and canyons throughout the Santa Ana Mountains. Within the Orange County area, the indicator tree is the live oak, but sycamores may also be abundantly present. In the Chino Hills, native walnut trees form a major component of the southern oak woodland community. Beneath the trees themselves, various chaparral and sage-scrub plants often form a sparse understory.

Aside from these three widespread natural communities, much of the non-urbanized land in and around Orange County is given over to agriculture and grazing. In areas characterized by heavy grazing, one finds grassy flats and bald slopes called *potreros* (pastures) supporting mostly nonnative grasses and herbs like wild oats, filaree, mustard, and fennel.

Several other natural communities of small extent are found in Orange County: *rocky shore, coastal strand, coastal salt marsh, freshwater marsh, riparian woodland, and coniferous forest.*

The riparian (streamside) woodland community, existing in discontinuous strips along some of the bigger watercourses, is perhaps the most biologically valuable. Not only is this kind of environment essential for the continued survival of many kinds of birds and animals; it is also very appealing to the senses. Massive sycamores, cottonwoods, and live oaks, and a screen of water-hugging willows are the hallmarks of the riparian woodland. Most of this habitat has already been usurped by urbanization and by the development of water resources.

The coniferous (cone-bearing tree) forest community was once more widespread in the Santa Ana Mountains. The west-side canyons were logged a century ago in connection with various short-lived mining booms; this logging and subsequent wildfires have reduced the forest to small, isolated patches that cling to the slopes of the deeper canyons. Big-cone Douglas-fir and Coulter pine are the indicator species of coniferous forest in the Santa Anas, although live oaks and other broadleaf trees are also frequently present.

A few species of plants of limited geographic extent in Orange County are worth noting:

Knobcone pine, somewhat widely distributed in the northern and central California Coast Ranges and the foothills of the Sierra Nevada, clings to a small toehold in the Santa Ana Mountains on the slopes of Pleasants Peak. Here it finds the warm, dry climate and the particular kind of soil—serpentine—it thrives on.

Bigleaf maple, California bay (bay laurel), and madrone, found in the west-side canyons of the Santa Ana Mountains, are three more examples of trees at or close to the southern end of their natural range. The madrones are restricted to a tiny area in upper Trabuco Canyon.

The Tecate cypress, once widespread throughout Southern California, is now confined to small "arboreal islands" in San Diego County, in northern Baja California, and along the slopes of Coal and Gypsum canyons in the northern Santa Anas (just outside the Cleveland Forest boundary). Here it finds the extra moisture, in the form of nocturnal fogs moving in from the coast, it needs in order to cling to its biological niche.

Late winter to mid-spring is the best time to appreciate the cornucopia of Orange County's native plants. Many of the showiest species—the annual wildflowers—burgeon at this time, and other plants exhibit fresh, new growth. For more information about the wildflowers, shrubs, trees, and other flora typically found in Orange County, see Appendix 3.

Creatures Great and Small

One's first sighting of an eagle, a mountain lion, a badger, or any other seldom-seen form of wildlife is always a memorable experience. Because of the diversity of the still-natural parts of Orange County, they are host to a healthy population of indigenous creatures, including a few rare and endangered species. If you're willing to stretch your legs a bit and spend some time in the areas favored by wild animals, you'll eventually be rewarded by some kind of close visual contact.

While doing field work for this book, I was lucky to spot a young mountain lion while hiking in the Santa Ana Mountains, and a golden eagle while driving on Interstate 5 through the hills of south county.

The most numerous large creature in Orange County is the mule deer, with a population of perhaps several hundred. These deer prefer areas of forest and chaparral, especially at higher elevations in the Santa Anas.

The mountain lion, once hunted to near-extinction in California, has made a comeback as a protected species. Perhaps two dozen lions now roam the remote canyons of the Santa Ana Mountains and foothill areas. Counting is difficult, since mountain lions have a large territorial range (up to 100 square miles) and are normally very secretive. Because of their wide-ranging travels, however, tracks and other signs of the mountain lion are quite frequently seen.

The county's mammals also include the coyote, which has adapted to a broad range of habitats, including the margins of suburbia; the bobcat, a creature sometimes mistaken for a mountain lion, but smaller and more common; the gray fox; the skunk; the opossum; the raccoon; the ringtail cat; the badger; and various rabbits, squirrels, bats, woodrats, and mice.

Among the more commonly seen reptiles are rattlesnakes, which I will discuss in the next section.

The richness of bird life in the Orange County area is impressive, not only because of the diversity of its habitats, but also because the county lies along the Pacific Flyway route of spring-fall bird migration and serves as a wintering area for waterfowl. Several species of rare or endangered birds nest or visit, including the southern bald eagle, the peregrine falcon, the lightfooted clapper rail, the least tern, the Belding's savannah sparrow, and the least Bell's vireo.

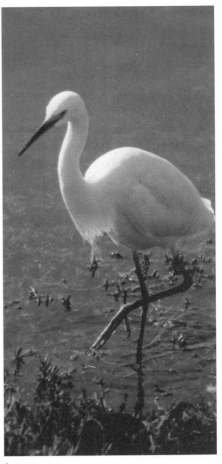

Snowy egret

Health, Safety and Courtesy

Good preparation is always important for any kind of recreational pursuit. Hiking Southern California's backcountry is no exception. Although most of our local environments are seldom hostile or dangerous to life and limb, there are some pitfalls to be aware of.

Preparation and Equipment

An obvious safety requirement is being in good health. Some degree of physical conditioning is always desirable, even for those trips in this book designated as easy or moderate. The more challenging trips (rated "moderately strenuous" or "strenuous" in difficulty) require stamina and occasionally some technical expertise. Fast walking, running, bicycling, swimming, aerobic dancing, and any similar exercise that develops both the leg muscles and the aerobic capacity of the whole body are recommended as preparatory exercise.

For long trips over rough trails or cross-country terrain (there are several of these in this book) there is no really adequate way to prepare other than practicing the activity itself. Start with easy- or moderate-length trips first to accustom the leg muscles to the peculiar stresses involved in walking over uneven terrain and scrambling over boulders, and to acquire a good sense of balance. As I will note later, hiking boots rather than lightweight shoes are preferred for such travel, primarily from a safety standpoint.

Since all hiking in the Orange County area is below 6000 feet elevation, health complications due to high altitude are rare. You may, however, notice some loss of energy and more rapid breathing in the higher parts of the Santa Ana Mountains.

An important aspect of preparation is the choice of equipment and supplies. The essentials you should carry with you at all times into the backcountry are the items that would allow you to survive, in a reasonably comfortable manner, one or two unscheduled nights out on the trail. It's important to note that no one ever plans these nights! No one plans to get lost, injured, stuck, or pinned down by the weather. Always do a "what if" analysis for a worst-case scenario, and plan accordingly. These essential items are your safety net; keep them with you on all your hikes.

Chief among the essential items is warm clothing. Away from the coast, winter temperatures can plummet from warm at midday to subfreezing at night. Layer your clothing: it is better to take along two or more middleweight outer garments than rely on a single heavy or bulky jacket to keep you comfortable at all times. Add to this a cap, gloves, and a waterproof or water-resistant shell (a large trash bag with a hole for your head will do in a pinch) and you'll be quite prepared for all but the most severe weather experienced in the areas described in this book.

In hot, sunny weather, sun-shielding clothing is another "essential." This would normally include a sun hat and a light-colored, long-sleeved top.

Water, and to a lesser extent, food are next in importance. If potable water isn't immediately available, carry a generous supply. On a hot summer's day in the Santa Anas, you might need to drink up to a gallon of water on a 10-mile hike. Food is needed to stave off hunger and keep energy stores up, but it is not as essential as water in a survival situation.

Down the list further, but still "essential," are a map and compass (or a GPS unit and the knowledge of its use); flashlight; fire-starting devices (examples: waterproof matches or lighter, and candle); and first-aid kit.

Items not always essential, but potentially very useful and convenient, are sunglasses, pocket knife, whistle (or other signaling device), sunscreen, and toilet paper.

The essential items mentioned above should be carried by every member of a hiking party, because individuals or splinter groups may end up separating from the party for one reason or another. If you plan to hike solo in the backcountry, being well-equipped is all-important. Be sure to check in with a park ranger or leave your itinerary with some other responsible person. In that way, if you do get stuck, help will probably come to the right place—eventually.

Special Hazards

Other than getting lost or pinned down by a rare sudden storm, the three most common hazards in the foothill and mountain areas are poison oak, ticks, and rattlesnakes. Poison oak, in bush or vine form, is common along many hillsides and canyons below 5000 feet. It often grows thickly on the banks of streamcourses, where it seems to prefer the semi-shade of live and scrub oaks. Learn to recognize its distinctive three-leafed structure, and avoid touching it with skin or clothing. Poison oak is deciduous, losing its leaves usually in summer or fall, but the bare stems are no guarantee of safety: the stems continue to harbor some of the toxic resin. If there's no avoiding contact with the poison oak plant, thick pants, such as jeans, and a long-sleeved shirt will serve as fair barriers for protecting your skin. Remove these clothes as soon as the hike is over, and make sure they are washed carefully afterward. Take a bath or shower as soon as possible.

Ticks can sometimes be the scourge of overgrown trails in the Santa Ana Mountains, particularly in mid-spring when they climb to the tips of shrub branches and lie in wait for warm-blooded hosts. Ticks are especially abundant along trails used by cattle, deer, and coyotes. If you can't avoid brushing against vegetation along the trail, be sure to check for ticks frequently. Upon finding a host, a tick will usually crawl upward some distance in search of a protected spot, where it will try to attach itself. If you're aware of the slightest irritation on your body, you'll be able to intercept the tick long before it attempts to bite.

Rattlesnakes are fairly common in brushy, rocky and streamside habitats from coast to mountains. Seldom seen in either cold or very hot weather, they favor temperatures in the 75–90° range. Expect to see (or hear) rattlesnakes out and about in the daytime from early spring to mid-fall, and at night in summer and early fall. Most rattlesnakes are every bit as interested in avoiding contact with you as you are with them. Watch carefully where you put your feet, and especially your hands, during rattlesnake season. In brushy or rocky areas where sight distance is short, try to make your presence known from afar. Tread with heavy footfalls, or use a stick to bang against rocks or bushes. Rattlesnakes will pick up the vibrations through their skin and will usually buzz (unmistakably) before you get too close for comfort.

Here are a few more safety tips:

Most free-flowing water should be regarded as unsafe for drinking without purification. This does not include, of course, developed water sources within campgrounds and picnic areas. Chemical (iodine or chlorine) treatment and filtering are the most convenient purification methods, but secondary in effectiveness to boiling. A bigger problem, of course, is the availability of the water itself. Many springs and watercourses in the Santa Anas are intermittent, flowing only after winter rains. Your best bet is to carry all the water you'll need on the trail.

Deer-hunting season in Cleveland National Forest occurs during mid-autumn. Although conflicts between hunters and hikers are not common, you may want to confine your explorations at that time of year to state and county parks, where hunting is prohibited.

Mountain lions do frequent the wilder corners of Orange County and have even been spotted on the edge of suburban neighborhoods. While recent news stories have trumpeted every instance of encounters with mountain lions, attacks on hikers or mountain bikers remain statistically rare. The following precautions are urged for all persons entering mountain lion country:

- Hike with one or more companions.

- Keep children close at hand.

- Never run from a mountain lion. This may trigger an instinct to attack.

- Make yourself "large," face the animal, maintain eye contact with it, shout, blow a whistle, and do not act fearful. Do anything to convince the animal that you are not its prey.

- Carry a hiking stick and use it, or pitch stones or other objects at the animal if it continues to advance.

There is always some risk in leaving a vehicle unattended at a remote trailhead. Fortunately automobile vandalism and burglary are not acute problems in the areas described in this book. Report all theft and vandalism of personal property to park officials or the county sheriff, and report vandalism of public property to the appropriate park or forest agency.

Trail Courtesy

Whenever you travel the backcountry wilderness, or even a well-trodden park trail, you take on a burden of responsibility to preserve the natural environment. Aside from common-sense prohibitions against littering and vandalism, there are some less obvious guidelines every hiker should be aware of. We'll mention a few:

Never cut trail switchbacks. This practice breaks down the trail tread and hastens erosion. Improve designated trails by removing branches, rocks, or other debris if you can. Report any trail damage and misplaced or broken signs to the appropriate ranger office (Cleveland National Forest has a form for this purpose).

When backpacking, be a "no trace" camper. Camp well away from water and leave your campsite as you found it or leave it in an even more natural condition. Because of the danger of wildfire, you cannot have open fires (campfires, barbecues) except in developed campgrounds and picnic grounds. For cooking, you can use a camp stove (with the proper permit), but only in an area cleared of flammable vegetation.

Collecting minerals, plants, animals, and historical objects without special permit is prohibited in state and county parks, and in the National Forest. This means common things, too, such as pine cones, wildflowers, and lizards. These should be left for all visitors to enjoy.

It is impractical to review here all the specific rules associated with the use of public lands in the Orange County area, but you, as a visitor, are responsible for knowing them. Refer to Appendix 5 for sources of information.

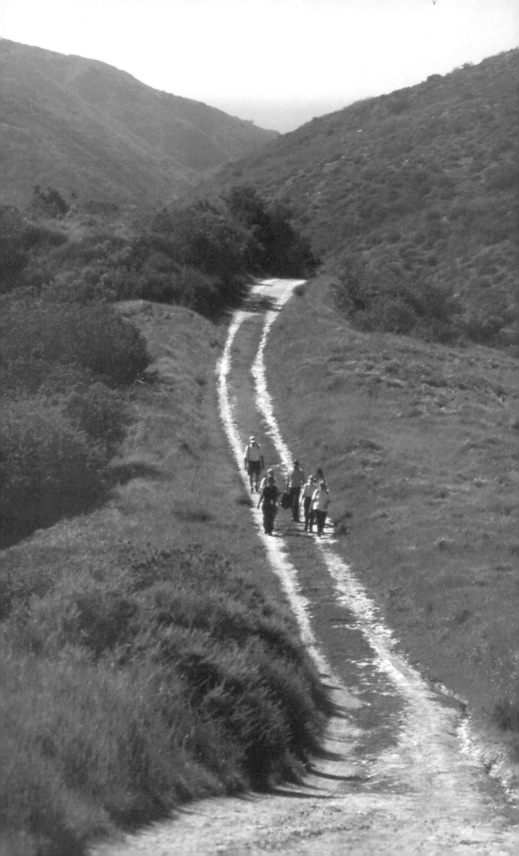

Using This Book

Whether you wish to use this book as a reference tool or as a guide to be read cover to cover, you should take a few minutes to read this section. Herein I explain the exact meaning of the capsulized information that appears before each trip description, and also describe the way in which trips are grouped together geographically.

One way to expedite the process of finding a suitable trip, especially if you're unfamiliar with hiking opportunities in Orange County, is to turn to Appendix 1, "Best Hikes." This is a cross reference of the most highly recommended hikes described in this book.

Each of the 87 hiking trips belongs to one of 14 geographical areas, which are organized as chapters in this book. Each chapter has its own introductory text and map. The chapters are grouped according to "regions" in and around Orange County. Chapters 1–5 cover the beaches, bays, and coastal plains of Orange County. Chapters 6–11 cover the foothills surrounding the Santa Ana Mountains. Chapters 12–14 cover the Santa Ana Mountains—more precisely, the Trabuco District of Cleveland National Forest, which encompasses the Santa Ana Mountains.

The index map of Orange County and vicinity (on pages vi and vii) shows the coverage of each chapter map, and the Table of Contents shows the page numbers for each region, chapter, and trip.

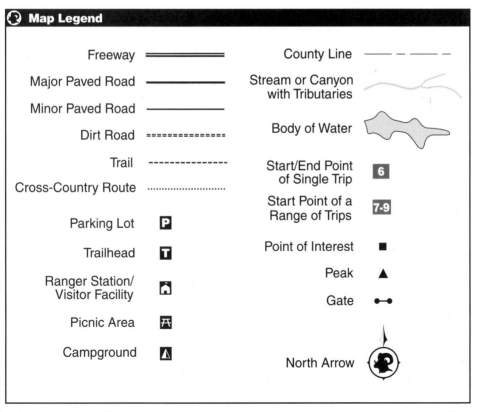

Map Legend

Freeway	County Line
Major Paved Road	Stream or Canyon with Tributaries
Minor Paved Road	
Dirt Road	Body of Water
Trail	Start/End Point of Single Trip **6**
Cross-Country Route	Start Point of a Range of Trips **7-9**
Parking Lot **P**	Point of Interest ■
Trailhead **T**	Peak ▲
Ranger Station/ Visitor Facility	Gate •—•
Picnic Area	
Campground	North Arrow

The introductory text for each chapter includes any general information about the area's history, geology, plants, and wildlife not included in the trip descriptions. Important information about possible restrictions or special requirements (wilderness permits, for example) appears here too, and you should review this material before starting on a hike in a particular chapter. In particular, you should be aware that nearly all trips on Cleveland National Forest land (nearly all the hikes in Chapters 12–14) require that you post a "National Forest Adventure Pass" on your parked car. For more information on this fee collection system, see the introductory section of Chapter 12, Santa Ana Mountains—Main Divide.

Each chapter also contains a sketch map of the locations and routes of all hikes in the area covered by that chapter. The numbers in the squares on those maps correspond to trip numbers in the text. These boxed numbers refer to the start/end points of out-and-back and loop trips. The point-to-point trips have two boxed numbers, indicating separate start and end points. For some hikes, the corresponding chapter map alone is complete enough and fully adequate for navigation; for other hikes, more detailed topographical or other maps are recommended. A legend for the maps appears on page 13.

Capsulized Information

The following is an explanation of the capsulized information appearing at the beginning of each trip description. If you are simply browsing through this book, these summaries alone can be used as a tool to eliminate from consideration hikes that are either too difficult or too trivial for your abilities or desires.

DISTANCE

An estimate of total distance is given. Out-and-back trips show the sum of the distances of the out and back segments. After the trail distance, I've noted whether the trip, as described, is a loop, an out-and-back route, or a point-to-point trip, requiring a car shuttle. There is some flexibility, of course, in the way in which a hiker can actually follow the trip.

HIKING TIME

This figure is for the average hiker, and includes only the time spent in motion. It does not include time spent for rest stops, lunch, etc. Fast walkers can complete the routes in perhaps 30% less time, and slower hikers may take 50% longer. The hiker is assumed to be traveling with a light day pack. (Important note: Do realize that "hiking time" stated in this book is for time-in-motion only. Also, hikers carrying heavy packs could easily take nearly twice as long, especially if they are traveling under adverse weather conditions. Remember, too, that the progress made by a group as a whole is limited by pace of the slowest member or members.)

ELEVATION GAIN/LOSS

This is an estimate of the sum of all the vertical gain segments and the sum of all the vertical loss segments along the total length of the route (includes both ways for out-and-back trips). This is often considerably more than the net difference in elevation between the high and low points of the hike.

DIFFICULTY

This overall rating takes into account the length of the trip and the nature of the terrain. The following are general definitions of the four categories:

EASY: Suitable for every member of the family.

MODERATE: Suitable for all physically fit people.

MODERATELY STRENUOUS: Long length, substantial elevation gain, and/or difficult terrain. Suitable for experienced hikers only.

STRENUOUS: Full day's hike (or overnight backpack) over a long and often difficult route. Suitable only for experienced hikers in excellent physical condition.

Each higher level represents more or less a doubling of the difficulty. On average, moderate trips are twice as hard as easy trips, moderately strenuous trips are twice as hard as moderate trips, and so on.

TRAIL USE

SUITABLE FOR BACKPACKING: Most trips in this book are not. Although there are several roadside campgrounds in the Orange County vicinity, trail camping is not widely permitted.

SUITABLE FOR MOUNTAIN BIKING: The route, as described, is open to mountain biking, and is reasonably safe for that activity. Since regulations governing the use of mountain bikes on trails may change, it is a good idea to check with the agency having jurisdiction over the area.

DOGS ALLOWED: This indicates that dogs are allowed on the trail, generally on a leash no longer than 6 feet.

GOOD FOR KIDS: These trips are especially recommended for inquisitive children. They were chosen on the basis of their safety and ease of travel, and their potential for entertaining the whole family.

BEST TIMES

Nearly all the short trips in this book are suitable year round, but some of the longer trips, especially those inland, are much more rewarding when temperatures are mild and/or water is present along the trail.

AGENCY

These code letters refer to the agency or office that has jurisdiction or management over the area being hiked (for example, CNF/TD means Cleveland National Forest, Trabuco District). You can contact the agency for more information. Full names, phone numbers, and some addresses (of larger agencies) are listed in Appendix 5.

OPTIONAL/RECOMMENDED MAP(S)

The topographic maps listed are nearly all U.S. Geological Survey 7.5-minute series topographic maps. Usually, these are the most complete and accurate maps of the physical features (if not always the cultural features and trails) of the area you'll be traveling in. These maps are typically stocked by backpacking, outdoor sports, and map shops around Southern California. Topographic maps on CD format and topographic-map images downloadable from the internet are becoming popular alternatives to purchasing hard-copy topographic maps. The state and regional parks in and around Orange County have done an excellent job of providing hiking maps at park entrances and trailheads. Topographic maps, however, are especially useful for hiking on Cleveland National Forest lands in the Santa Ana Mountains.

NOTES

Only one of these three terrain designations appears in the "Notes" section for a given trip, indicating the general character of the terrain encountered. Light footwear (running or walking shoes) is appropriate for easy terrain, while sturdy hiking boots are recommended for more difficult terrain

EASY TERRAIN: roads, trails, and easy cross-country hiking

MODERATE TERRAIN: cross-country boulder hopping and easy scrambling

DIFFICULT TERRAIN: nontechnical climbing required (Warning: These trips should be attempted only by suitably equipped, experienced hikers adept at traveling over steep or rocky terrain requiring the use of the hands as well as the feet.)

Nontechnical climbing includes everything up to Class 3 on the rock climber's scale. While ropes and climbing hardware are not required, a hiker should have a good sense of balance, and enough experience to recognize dangerous moves and situations. The safety and stability of hiking boots are especially recommended for this kind of trip. Hazards may include loose or slippery rocks and rattlesnakes (don't put your hands in places you can't see clearly).

"Bushwhacking" indicates cross-country travel through dense brush is required. I have noted this when trips require a substantial amount of off-trail "bushwhacking." Wear long pants and be especially alert for rattlesnakes

Only one of these two designations appears in the "Notes" section: "Marked Trails/Obvious Routes" or "Navigation Required" (Warning: Trips for which navigation skills are required should be attempted only by hikers skilled in navigation techniques and map and compass or GPS use.)

Unambiguous cross-country routes up a canyon, for example, are noted as having "Marked Trails/Obvious Routes". The hiker, of course, should never be without a map in any remote area, even if there are marked trails or the route seems obvious.

Old mining trail above Santiago Canyon

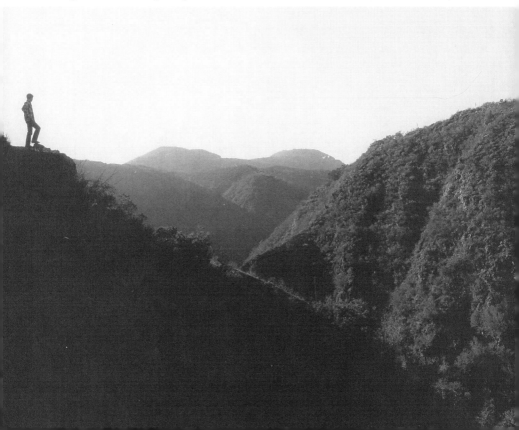

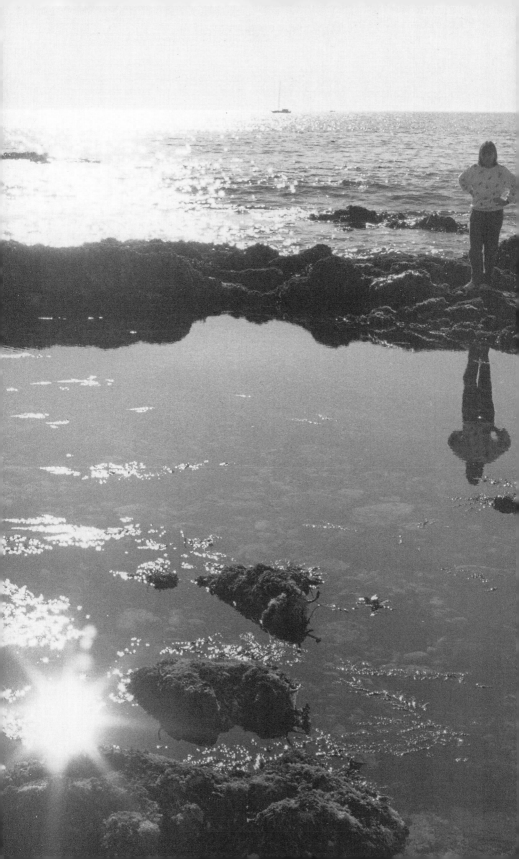

Chapter 1

Beaches and Bays:
North Coast

Orange County's northernmost stretch of coastline consists of a wide, sandy strand stretching through the cities of Seal Beach and Huntington Beach. Tens of thousands of people flock to these beaches on warm, sunny days, while tens of thousands more live immediately back of the coastline on low-lying land that once supported extensive salt-water and fresh-water marshes.

The underlying sedimentary rocks are rich in petroleum; you're reminded of that by the sight of rocker pumps, storage tanks, and refineries. That activity, however, is waning. New housing developments are springing up, especially

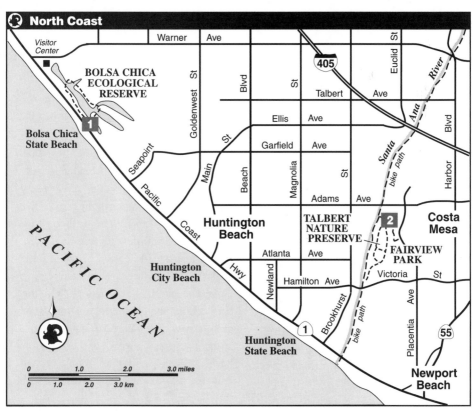

North Coast

Visitor Center

Warner Ave

405

Euclid St

Ana River

BOLSA CHICA ECOLOGICAL RESERVE

Goldenwest St

Blvd

St

Talbert Ave

Ellis Ave

Bolsa Chica State Beach

1

St

Garfield Ave

Seapoint

Main St

Beach St

Magnolia St

Adams Ave

Santa

bike path

Blvd

Harbor

Pacific

Coast

Huntington Beach

TALBERT NATURE PRESERVE

2

Costa Mesa

Atlanta Ave

FAIRVIEW PARK

Victoria St

PACIFIC OCEAN

Huntington City Beach

Hwy

Newland

Hamilton Ave

Brookhurst

bike path

Ave

Placentia Ave

55

1

1

Huntington State Beach

Newport Beach

0   1.0   2.0   3.0 miles
0   1.0   2.0   3.0 km

Little Corona tidepool (see Chapter 3)

along the Pacific Coast Highway. Formerly environmentally abused wetlands and floodplains are in the process of being restored to some semblance of an original condition.

Two areas along this north stretch of coast stand out as excellent examples of ecological rehabilitation: Bolsa Chica Ecological Reserve and Talbert Nature Preserve. Both are perfect for easy-going exercise and early-morning bird and wildlife watching. Huntington Beach boasts of being one of the nation's best birding sites, with nearly half of all birds in the nation spotted there. The prevalance of hikers and birdwatchers with elaborate spotting scopes and telephoto lenses at Bolsa Chica and other nearby coastal locales attests to that.

TRIP 1 Bolsa Chica Ecological Reserve

Distance	1.5 miles, Loop
Hiking Time	1 hour
Difficulty	Easy
Trail Use	Good for kids
Best Times	All year
Agency	BCER
Optional Map	USGS 7.5-min *Seal Beach*
Notes	Marked trails/obvious routes, easy terrain

DIRECTIONS The Bolsa Chica Ecological Reserve trailhead lies on the inland side of Pacific Coast Highway, 1.5 miles south of Warner Avenue, and 1.5 miles north of Seapoint Avenue in Huntington Beach.

The noisy coast highway and may put you off a bit, but don't let that deter you from trying this pathway around Bolsa Chica Slough. Binoculars, spotting scopes, and/or cameras are de rigueur, of course.

First, consider paying a visit to the Bolsa Chica Interpretive Center on Warner Avenue at Pacific Coast Highway. A checklist of local birds and information about the reserve can be obtained there.

From the parking lot a long, wooden bridge leads over some shallow stretches of tide water invaded by typical saltwater marsh plants: cordgrass, alkali heath, sea lavender, and pickleweed. Interpretive panels tell of two endangered species of birds that frequent this area: the least tern, which nests on two small, sandy islands nearby; and the Belding's savannah sparrow, a bird that can drink sea water, processing it with hyper-efficient kidneys. Early on weekend mornings, photographers use the bridge as a stable platform for their often sophisticated equipment.

On the far side of the bridge a path goes left atop a levee, eventually encircling a segment of the slough. On the surface and the shoreline you may spot gulls, terns, egrets, cormorants, pelicans, stilts, plovers, avocets, grebes, marsh hawks, herons, and kites. The number and diversity of birds vary with the season.

At one point along the way, you can walk up to a scenic viewpoint on the lip of a nearby mesalike terrace. Gabrieleno Indians contemplated a lonely scene here centuries ago. They beheld a broad, shallow bay extending well inland, rimmed by salt- and fresh-water marshes as far as the eye could see.

Note: A major restoration project was underway here at the time of this writing, and the loop trail was temporarily closed. The goal of this work, which may be completed in 2007, is to return 550 acres of Bolsa Chica marsh and lowland to its pre-1900 condition. In less than a decade, the odiferous and unsightly oil-drilling site adjoining the slough will have been transformed into a scenic treasure and a major wildlife stopover for millions of migrating birds.

Bolsa Chica Slough

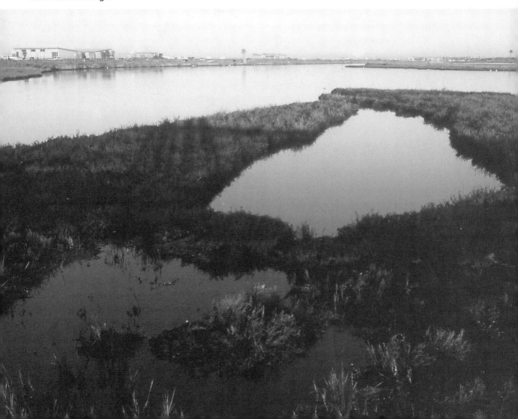

TRIP 2 Talbert Nature Preserve

Distance	2 miles or more, Loop
Hiking Time	1 hour
Difficulty	Easy
Trail Use	Dogs allowed, mountain biking allowed, good for kids
Best Times	All year
Agency	TNP
Optional Map	USGS 7.5-min *Seal Beach*
Notes	Marked trails/obvious routes, easy terrain

DIRECTIONS The starting point is Fairview Park on the western edge of the city of Costa Mesa. Drive to the park's main entrance on the west side of Placentia Avenue, 0.5 mile south of Adams Avenue, and 1.0 mile north of Victoria Street.

Another large restoration project has been in progress in recent years along the flood plain just east of the channelized Santa Ana River in the city of Costa Mesa. Talbert Nature Preserve consists of two sections divided by busy Victoria Street: a north part laced with wide, smooth trails, and a south part still undergoing major restoration.

The planting of native vegetation in the preserve is being guided both by remaining native vegetation on site and by attempts to recreate plant communities similar to those that existed in this region before nearly every available acre was put to use for agriculture, housing, or industry. Several plant "zones" in the preserve are identified here by means of trailside interpretive plaques. The zones include coastal strand, native grassland, alluvial woodland, and wetland vegetation. Thus the preserve serves as a native

Talbert Nature Preserve

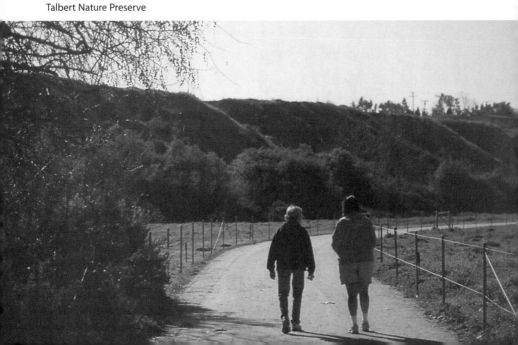

botanical garden, a refuge for wildlife, an educational resource, and a recreational resource.

From the restrooms near the main entrance to Fairview Park, walk a short distance west, and turn right on the paved bike path. Follow the path north and then west down a hill until you reach the Talbert Nature Preserve's entrance on the left, which is marked by a dome-shaped restroom building and an information kiosk. (The paved path itself continues west to a tie-in with the Santa Ana River bike path, which suggests another way to reach Talbert's entrance if you are arriving by bicycle.)

A wide, flat, decomposed-granite path suitable for hikers, cyclists and horses runs toward the south from the entrance for a short mile, beneath the brow of a steep bluff. It then connects with a segment of paved bike path leading to Victoria Street. Short of that juncture, there are opportunities to branch west and loop back to the entrance using unimproved trails. Those alternate trails may turn muddy after significant rainfall.

I found Talbert Nature Preserve to be an extraordinarily quiet place, effectively screened from traffic noise by the bluff rising on the east and levees on west which effectively deaden the din from the surrounding cityscape.

Chapter 2

Beaches and Bays:
Upper Newport Bay

The marshes surrounding Upper Newport Bay represent tiny remnants of a much more extensive wetland that once stretched inland to the present city of Tustin. The Portola expedition of 1769 and subsequent travelers passing up- or down-coast avoided this soggy region and stuck to the base of the foothills, where the firm ground more than made up for the inconvenience of traversing ridges and ravines.

During the past 100,000 years or more the Santa Ana River has wandered across the surface of the Los Angeles Basin, changing course many times in response to flooding and silt deposition. Around

Matilija poppy

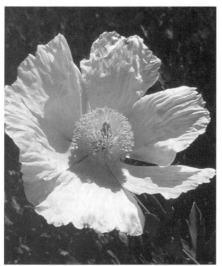

30,000 years ago, the river (which at that time carried more runoff because of a wetter climate) carved out the basic form of the trough-like structure now occupied by Upper Newport Bay. Sediment carried by the river and dropped at the mouth of the trough formed a barrier island, today's Balboa Peninsula, enclosing (lower) Newport Bay.

The most recent natural shift in the Santa Ana River's course occurred in 1825, when a large flood redirected the flow west from Upper Newport Bay to essentially the place where it reaches the ocean today via artificial channel. Today the bay is fed by San Diego Creek, a small former tributary of the river.

For many millennia decayed marsh vegetation (peat) accumulated along the upper bay shores. This material, mixed with fine silt washed down from the surrounding slopes and bluffs, has created the kind of soil conditions conducive to self-sustaining wetlands.

Hemmed in by bustling traffic arteries, high-rise office buildings, residential areas, and the Irvine campus of the University of California, Upper Newport Bay exists in a kind of time warp. Coyotes and mule deer still roam the periphery, while myriads of migratory birds use the productive marshes as a stopover or a winter home.

The future of the wetlands around Upper Newport Bay has been assured by the establishment of three protected areas. One of them, the Upper Newport Bay Ecological Reserve encompasses most of the bay's salt-water marshes. Just upstream along the channelized San Diego Creek are two more areas, protect-ing only a fraction of the freshwater marsh that once extended inland for sev-eral miles. Some 200 acres of the marsh became U.C. Irvine's San Joaquin Fresh-water Marsh Reserve in 1970. That facil-ity is now being managed as a research reserve accessible only to qualified researchers. The adjacent and much

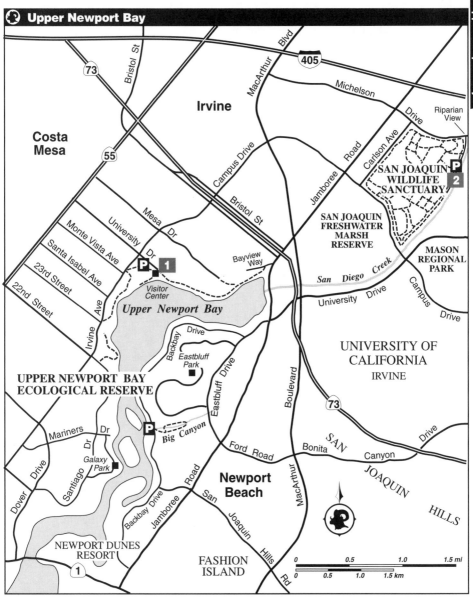

newer San Joaquin Wildlife Sanctuary, on the other hand, has been designed for extensive use by recreational users and amateur naturalists. An amazing 10 miles of wide, smoothly graded trails crisscross the wildlife sanctuary, which covers 300 acres of diked ponds, natural riparian habitat, and artificially created native habitats.

TRIP 1 Upper Newport Bay Ecological Reserve

Distance	Various walks up to 1 mile
Hiking Time	Varies
Difficulty	Easy
Trail Use	Dogs allowed, suitable for mountain biking, good for kids
Best Times	All year
Agency	UNBER
Optional Maps	USGS 7.5-min *Newport Beach, Tustin*
Notes	Marked trails/obvious routes, easy terrain

DIRECTIONS To reach Upper Newport Bay's interpretive center, exit the Costa Mesa Freeway (Highway 55) at Del Mar Avenue in Costa Mesa, and go east toward the bay. In ½ mile, Del Mar becomes University Drive. Continue a short distance past Irvine Avenue to reach the interpretive center parking lot. There's convenient access to most of the existing bayside trails from here.

Were it not for public protest in the 1960s and '70s, Upper Newport Bay would surely have become yet another of Orange County's residential harbor communities. Instead, the State of California purchased 752 acres of Irvine Company land in 1975, thus establishing the Upper Newport Bay Ecological Reserve.

An astounding 100 species of coastal and mudflat fish frequent the shallow waters of the bay, as well as some 200 species of birds. To appreciate the reserve, most people drive, bike, jog, or walk along Backbay Drive on the east shore. Backbay Drive is one-way north for cars.

At about the halfway point along the Backbay Drive, at the mouth of Big Canyon, there's an interpretive display and shoreline view point on the west side, and short trail/boardwalk visiting a small freshwater marsh on the east side.

The north shore features a bayshore bikeway connecting Bayview Way with the west segment of University Drive. At one point you pass over a massively timbered wood bridge spanning the marsh where it pinches against a steep, dry bluff. From that bridge you can view three separate tiers of vegetation. The lowest is the usual low-growing, salt-tolerant group of plants like pickleweed and cordgrass. Just above the reach of the tide are plants typical of the coastal uplands, such as wild buckwheat, mulefat, and cattails. Above the level of the bridge, the bluff slope supports a dense growth of native coastal sage-scrub vegetation: California sagebrush, lemonade berry, elderberry, prickly pear cactus, and cholla cactus (a coastal variant of the same cactus that grows abundantly throughout the California and Southwest deserts).

Upper Newport Bay's new interpretive center nuzzles into the ground near the corner of Irvine Avenue and University Drive, and a couple of short trails descend from there to the bay shoreline. A new interpretive trail meanders on the edge of the bluff just east of Irvine Avenue between 23rd Street and Monte Vista Avenue.

Finally, an unimproved trail on the west shore starts at the dead-end of a short residential street, Constellation Drive, off Santiago Drive, just east of the intersection of Irvine Avenue and 22nd Street. The path descends to the shoreline, curves north, and basically peters out in a grove of trees.

From most places along the west shore there's a good view of the broad sweep of the bay's channels and marshy islands, the steep bluffs rising from the far (east)

shore, and the rolling San Joaquin Hills beyond. Incised into the roughly 10-million-year-old marine sedimentary cliffs on the far side is a canyon that contained the largest assemblage of invertebrate fossils ever found in western North America.

From sea level to their highest summits, the San Joaquin Hills exhibit eight distinct marine-terrace levels. You may recognize some of these, though massive grading for construction has greatly altered the natural contour of the land. During excavation for the Fashion Island shopping center at Newport Center (cluster of high rises), a great deal of petrified wood was uncovered.

For an even broader view of the bay and surroundings, visit either Galaxy Park or Eastbluff Park in the nearby blufftop residential areas.

Freshwater marsh, Big Canyon

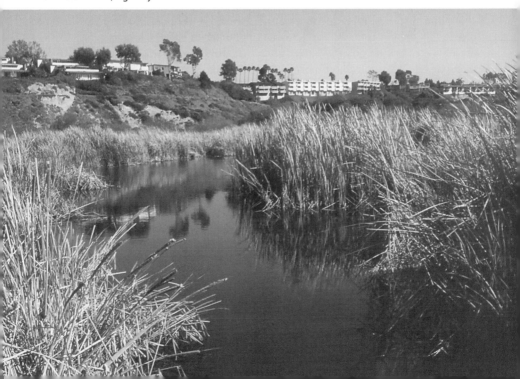

TRIP 2 San Joaquin Wildlife Sanctuary

Distance	Various walks up to several miles
Hiking Time	Varies
Difficulty	Easy to moderate
Trail Use	Good for kids
Best Times	All year
Agency	SJWS
Optional Map	USGS 7.5-min *Tustin*
Notes	Marked trails/obvious routes, easy terrain

DIRECTIONS Exit Interstate 405 at Jamboree Road. Go south about ⅓ mile to Michelson Drive. Turn left and continue 0.7 mile east to Riparian View on the right. Go a short distance south to either of two trailhead parking lots.

As one of the richest wetland areas along the Southern California coast, the San Joaquin Wildlife Sanctuary offers an uncommon opportunity to come in contact with a natural ecosystem seemingly plunked down in the midst of Orange County's high-rise urban core. Amid willows, cattails, and tules, you can spy on ducks, geese, and shorebirds, listen to bullfrog choruses, and perhaps even spot pond turtles sunning themselves on protruding limbs. You can thrill to the graceful antics of herons and egrets, and the soaring flights of the almost ever-present marsh hawks.

Make no mistake, the entire 300-acre spread, in its present incarnation, is essentially an urban park, planted densely with native trees and shrubs and irrigated with water from holding ponds that are a part of a state-of-the-art wastewater treatment plant. Starting in the 1990s, the Irvine Ranch Water District, with the support of the Irvine Company and the Sea and Sage chapter of the Audubon Society, began an ambitious project to transform the once neglected and raw-looking property into a naturalistic landscape typical of Orange County's original lowland and upland habitats. That effort, largely completed now, has resulted in a tightly nested system of more than 10 miles of wide, smooth, wheelchair-accessible trails, restrooms and resting benches galore, and most importantly a first-class habitat for birds.

Audubon volunteers have installed dozens of nestboxes throughout the sanctuary to attract cavity-nesting birds, and they conduct a monthly bird census which has resulted in sightings of nearly 300 species of birds to date.

A one-page free map available at both trailheads details the various designated hiking routes within the sanctuary.

The southern of the two trailheads on Riparian View marks the beginning of the 0.8-mile-long Tree Hill Trail, perhaps the best route for getting an overview of what the place has to offer. On it, you first visit Tree Hill, where African acacias and other exotic trees dot the top of a small knoll—a landscape demonstration project begun by the water district on Earth Day 1990. You then descend past planted pines, sycamores, and cottonwoods, and through a meticulously tended facsimile of sage-scrub and chaparral habitat. Curling around the perimeter of the water-treatment plant, you find yourself on the levee of one of the several rectangular ponds, which are actually settling basins.

The Tree Hill Trail "route" ends halfway around the first settling basin, but that's just the perfect place to start circling one or more of the five natural looking ponds (designated Ponds 1 through 5 on the trail map), which offer excellent opportunities for serendipitous discoveries of birds and other wildlife.

The San Joaquin Wildlife Sanctuary is clearly a place for wandering and quiet observation, rather than goal-oriented hiking. In fact, the whole place was carefully designed with berms, fences, and landscaping designed to screen out sight and sound of the surrounding city and its traffic.

Pond 4 at San Joaquin Wildlife Sanctuary

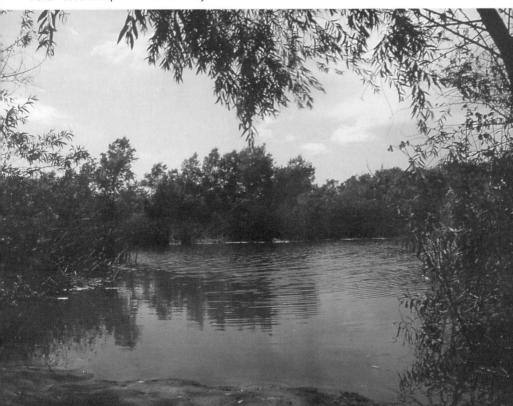

Chapter 3

Beaches and Bays:
Crystal Cove State Park

South of Newport Bay the shoreline topography, so flat and uninspiring back along the north county coast, becomes bold and dramatic. Cliffs provide a backdrop for restless surf breaking upon smooth, sandy beaches and rocky reefs, or surging into secluded coves. In the hills behind the wavecut cliffs, you can see, imprinted on the slopes, a muted stair-step pattern of earlier cliffs that used to be ocean-fronts long before this area was uplifted to its present height.

From Corona del Mar through the posh communities of Laguna Beach and Laguna Niguel to Dana Point, rustic cottages, opulent ocean-view homes, gated housing complexes, and swank hotels blanket most of the coastline. Interspersed with these thickly populated areas lie conspicuously blank areas on the street maps—sensuously curved hills and lush valleys that represent what nearly all of southern Orange County was like a century ago. Fortunately, some large pieces of the undeveloped land will never succumb to the ever-rising tide of suburbia. Over the past three decades, several large parcels of undeveloped land near

Sea stars

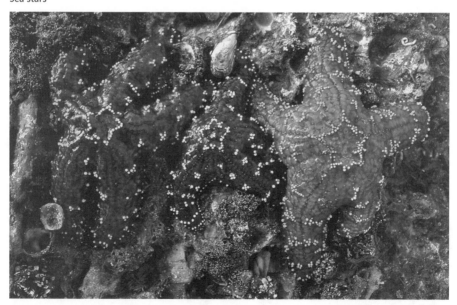

Laguna Beach have passed into public ownership.

Crystal Cove State Park was the first large parcel to be set aside. Besides a 3-mile stretch of bluffs and ocean front, the park reaches back into the San Joaquin Hills to encompass the entire watershed of El Moro Canyon—2200 acres of natural ravines, ridges, and terrace formations. In the backcountry (El Moro Canyon) section of the park alone, visitors can explore 18 miles of dirt roads and paths open to hikers, equestrians, and mountain bicyclists. Several more miles of paved bike path and trail lace the coastal blufftops and descend to the beach.

South and west of Crystal Cove State Park, several large parcels of undeveloped land in the San Joaquin Hills, owned for many decades by the Irvine Company, have passed into public ownership. These parcels, now incorporated into units called the Laguna Coast Wilderness Park and the Aliso and Wood Canyons Wilderness Park, are covered in Chapter 4, the Laguna Coast section of this book.

Crystal Cove State Park is open for day use from dawn to dusk. You can park along the beach and enjoy some tidepooling or beach-walking. Or you can drive up to the parking area adjoining the visitor center just east of Pacific Coast Highway, and start your exploration of the backcountry sector of the park from there. Mountain biking is both permitted and popular in Crystal Cove's backcountry section, not only on fire-road and former fire roads, but also on the narrow, "single-track" trails. This situation is

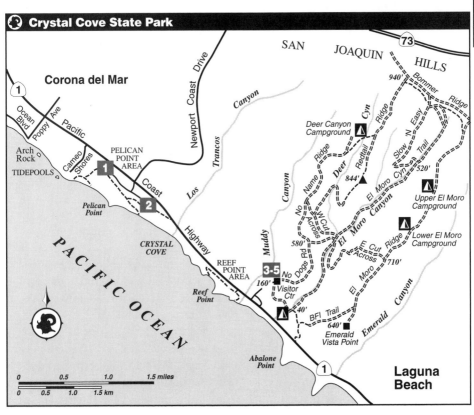

unusual for state parks, which often reserve the narrow trails for hiking use only.

At present there is no drive-in camping in Crystal Cove State Park, though plans for campground on the grounds of the present El Moro trailer park have long been afoot. At Crystal Cove itself, a historic cabin community is undergoing restoration for eventual short-term rentals for park visitors. Hike-in camping in the park is available at the Lower El Moro, Upper El Moro, and Deer Canyon trail camping sites.

The park's interpretive program includes occasional lectures and weekly outdoor activities such as bird-watching sessions, tidepool walks, and canyon hikes. As at any California state park, expect to pay a substantial parking fee for attending events or just exploring on your own. These fees go a long way toward maintaining the park's facilities and infrastructure, which are designed to accommodate heavy use.

TRIP 1 Corona Rock-hop

Distance	1 to 2 miles round trip, Out-and-back
Hiking Time	1 to 2 hours (round trip)
Elevation Gain/Loss	50'/50'
Difficulty	Moderate
Trail Use	Good for kids
Best Times	Low tide; October through March
Agency	CCSP
Optional Map	USGS 7.5-min *Laguna Beach*
Notes	Marked trails/obvious routes, moderate terrain

DIRECTIONS At the intersection of Pacific Coast Highway and Newport Coast Drive, south of Corona del Mar, turn west into Crystal Cove State Park (Pelican Point entrance). Bear right beyond the ranger hut to reach the northmost parking lot on the coastal bluff.

Some of the finest tidepools in Orange County—indeed in all of Southern California—await you on this short, absorbing, and probably time-consuming, rock-hopping trek between the Pelican Point area of Crystal Cove State Park and Little Corona City Beach in Corona del Mar. Wear an old pair of rubber-soled shoes or boots (boots are better for ankle support), and expect to get wet below the ankles. Don't turn your back to the incoming waves, otherwise you may get more wet than that.

Successful tidepool gazing requires both good light (midafternoon is best) and minus tides. These conditions are satisfied near the time of either new or full moon during the period from October through March. On about 20 afternoons each year, the tide drops to less than minus 1 foot, which is low enough for you to examine marine life at the lowermost intertidal zone. Plan to start your walk about an hour before predicted low tide.

Rocky reefs are exposed frequently along Crystal Cove State Park's beach-front, but not to the degree found along a 0.5-mile stretch of coast just north of the park.

From the Pelican Point parking area, a paved bike path—lined with native planted shrubs and spring wildflowers—swings toward the edge of the bluff. Soon there's a split: left toward the beach, right toward a viewpoint overlooking the ocean. For the rock-hopping trip, de-scend to the beach and turn up-coast over boulders and finlike rock formations into the tidepool area. The rock formations in the tidepools and the nearby cliffs are thinly bedded shales, gently tilted and sometimes fantastically contorted, dating back about 12 million years. In most but not all places in the intertidal zone, this

rock affords good traction even when wet.

On your way up toward Little Corona Beach you'll pass two picturesque sea stacks just offshore, both pierced by wave action. The northern of the two is named Arch Rock, but either could just as well have been called Bird Rock for the ever-present pelicans and other avian life.

In the intertidal strip itself, a few dozen steps from high-tide to low-tide level encompass a complete spectrum of marine plants and animals adapted to the various degrees of inundation and expo-sure. In the high intertidal zone, hardy species like periwinkle snails, limpets, mussels, barnacles, and green sea anemones are found. Some of these crea-tures are adapted to survival in habitats moistened only by the splash of breaking waves. Shore crabs patrol these bouldered

Crystal Cove State Park

Sea cave near Arch Rock

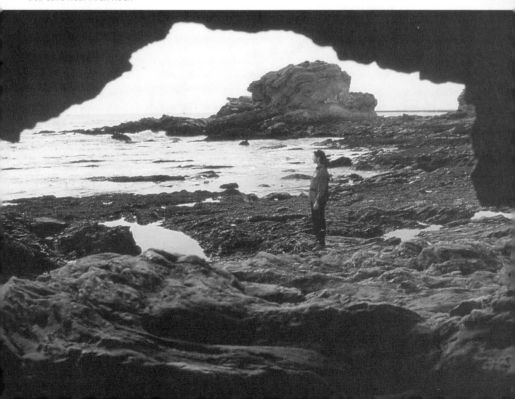

spaces, but they're likely to be hiding when you're looking for them.

Closer to the surf, the middle intertidal zone features the rock depressions called tidepools, and luxuriant growths of surfgrass, which look like bright, shiny green mats of long-bladed grass. The tidepools serve as refuges for mobile animals like fish, shrimp, and the sluglike sea hare, as well as some of the relatively immobile animals like urchins and various shellfish. Here the effects of biological erosion (or weathering) are apparent in the many pits and cubbyholes in the rocks occupied by various creatures.

In the low intertidal zone, many kinds of seaweeds thrive, including the intriguing sea palm. Animal life, however, is usually concealed beneath the rocks. Look for sea stars, sea urchins, sponges, worms, chitons, snails, abalones, and hermit crabs. If you're very lucky, an octopus may come your way. Remember that all marine life, shells, and rocks are protected.

Go as far as Little Corona Beach, and then return the same way you came.

TRIP 2 Crystal Cove Beaches

Distance	2 to 5 miles
Hiking Time	1 to 2 hours
Difficulty	Easy to moderate
Trail Use	Good for kids
Best Times	All year
Agency	CCSP
Optional Map	USGS 7.5-min *Laguna Beach*
Notes	Marked trails/obvious routes, easy terrain

DIRECTIONS There are three separate entrances to the bluff-and-beach section of Crystal Cove State Park. All entries are clearly marked with large, brown signs posted on Pacific Highway between Corona del Mar and Laguna Beach.

Hemmed in by hundred-foot cliffs on one side and the restless surf on the other, Crystal Cove State Park's 3 miles of sandy beachfront seem strangely detached from the busy world above. Aside from the quaint beachfront-cottage community at Crystal Cove, recognized on the National Register of Historic Places, the midportion of the beach is largely free of encroachment by human-made structures. Come early in the morning, or anytime on a cold or rainy day, and you may have the beach all to yourself.

The blufftops represent the first (other than the one being cut now at beach level) of several successively higher and older marine terraces extending back into the interior San Joaquin Hills. Stay on the designated paths so as not to trample the sage-scrub plant and wildlife community that has been reestablished here. Much of this vegetation looks brown and drab in the summer and fall months, when it is dormant, but it turns green and colorful during the rainy season.

The tops of the bluffs are excellent for watching the near-shore migration of gray whales from December through February. Using binoculars, scan the ocean surface out to a distance of 1 or 2 miles. Early- to mid-morning light (side-light) is best for this.

Below the cliffs on the gently shelving beach, you can scuff through the warm, squeaky sand above the high-tide line, tiptoe through the beached kelp along with flocks of nervous shorebirds, or cool off in the undulating wash of the surf. Swimmers and surfers should beware of the rocky reefs submerged at higher tides. During low tides, the rocky reefs are exposed, promising tidepool discoveries.

TRIP 3 Emerald Vista Point

Distance	5.0 miles, Loop
Hiking Time	2½ hours
Elevation Gain/Loss	900'/900'
Difficulty	Moderate
Trail Use	Suitable for mountain biking, suitable for backpacking, good for kids
Best Times	October through May
Agency	CCSP
Recommended Map	USGS 7.5-min *Laguna Beach;* or Crystal Cove State Park backcountry map
Notes	Marked trails/obvious routes, easy terrain

DIRECTIONS Crystal Cove State Park's visitor center and backcountry trailhead is located just east of Pacific Coast Highway, 2 miles north of Laguna Beach and 3 miles south of Corona del Mar. The entrance driveway is well marked, and a traffic light has been installed here for safety.

O n the most transparent winter days, the view from Emerald Vista Point spans more than 200 miles of Southern California coast and extends out to sea for a distance of 100 miles or more. Beyond Dana Point to the southeast, the low profile of San Diego's Point Loma can be traced along the curving shore-line, while offshore the diminutive Coro-nado Islands (just south of the international border) barely rise above the ocean haze. Southwest and west stand two big islands, San Clemente and Santa Catalina, the former a gently rising blister on the ocean surface, the latter a bold headland sprawling across 25 degrees of ocean horizon. Over the top of the upthrust Palos Verdes peninsula and through the often murky Los Angeles Basin to the northwest, you can some-times spy the Santa Monica Mountains and the faint blue coastline reaching west toward Santa Barbara.

Morning light is best for distant views, so plan an early start. From the entrance to the visitor center parking lot, take the wide trail leading south across a grassy flat. You soon begin a short, steep descent into the flat bottom of El Moro Canyon (0.4 mile), where you meet a wide, well traveled trail going up the canyon. On the right lies a trailer park that will be the site of the future El Moro drive-in campground. Turn left, heading up-canyon, then very quickly turn right on the narrow BFI Trail going up a grassy slope to the south. After gaining about 200 feet of elevation, you connect with a service road winding up the west spur of El Moro Ridge. Continue climbing up the service road for 0.7 mile, then make a sharp right on a spur leading south to a small antenna facility on the shoulder of the ridge. This is where views of Emerald Bay, the city of Laguna Beach, and the previously described distant ocean views are most panoramic.

For a longer, more leisurely descent, follow the service road farther north along El Moro Ridge (signed "Moro Ridge Road"), then veer left down the East Cut-Across road to El Moro Canyon. Turn left there and go down-canyon 1.0 mile to reach the wide trail leading out of the canyon and back toward the visitor center.

If you are backpacking, you'll be traveling farther north up El Moro Ridge. Add another 1.2 miles for the round trip to the Lower El Moro trail camp, or 2.8 miles round trip if you're heading to the Upper El Moro trail camp.

Afternoon view, Emerald Vista

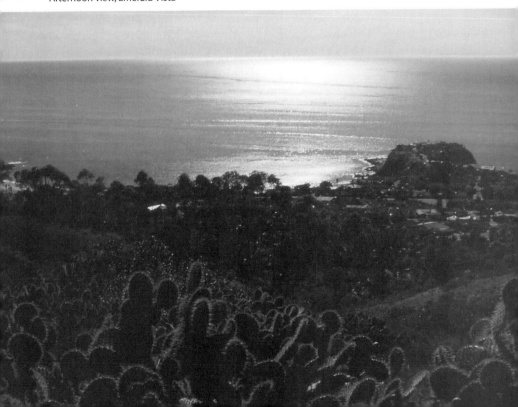

TRIP 4 El Moro Canyon Loop

Distance	8.3 miles, Loop
Hiking Time	5 hours
Elevation Gain/Loss	1400'/1400'
Difficulty	Moderately strenuous
Trail Use	Suitable for mountain biking
Best Times	October through May
Agency	CCSP
Recommended Map	USGS 7.5-min *Laguna Beach;* or Crystal Cove State Park backcountry map
Notes	Marked trails/obvious routes, easy terrain

DIRECTIONS Crystal Cove State Park's visitor center and backcountry trailhead is located just east of Pacific Coast Highway, 2 miles north of Laguna Beach and 3 miles south of Corona del Mar. The entrance driveway is well marked, and a traffic light has been installed here for safety.

On this grand, looping tour of the Crystal Cove backcountry you'll enjoy wide-ranging views from the spine of a prominent ridge along the way up, and admire upper El Moro Canyon's fine oak woodlands on the way back down.

From the visitor center parking lot take the dirt road leading east (No Dogs Road) toward a dry, scrub-covered ridge. After you climb a little, and if the morning marine-layer clouds have evaporated, nice views will open up of lower El Moro Canyon, the surrounding hills, and the blue ocean. Hawks and ravens soar on the updrafts generated on the sun-warmed slopes.

After 0.9 mile a powerline road on the right drops straight down into El Moro Canyon. Stay left and proceed generally north along the ridgeline. At the next intersection (1.5 miles) turn right on the West Cut-Across road. Descend only 0.2 mile, and then turn left on Rattlesnake Trail. Rattlesnake Trail contours around a steep ravine (Deer Canyon) then climbs to the nose of the ridge between El Moro and Deer canyons.

As you approach an 844-foot high point on the ridge, the hike takes on more of a wild character. The trail, now called Redtail Ridge Trail, narrows to footpath-width and passes delicately sculpted outcrops of sandstone. The native coastal sage-scrub vegetation crowding the trailside exudes a warm, spicy odor. In spring, the colorful blooms of sticky monkeyflower, goldenbush, and paintbrush play counterpoint to the muted greens of the sages, buckwheat, laurel sumac, and lemonade berry. Two kinds of cactus appear: common prickly pear cactus and the somewhat uncommon coast cholla cactus, whose easily detached bristling joints may snag the skin, clothing, or shoes of careless passersby.

At one point along the ridge, most of the near and far suburban landscapes are temporarily veiled from sight by intervening ridges, and for a moment you can picture southern Orange County as it was about a hundred years ago. On clear days, Mount San Antonio (Old Baldy) pokes up behind a nearby ridge to the north, and Santa Catalina Island seems to float

Crystal Cove State Park

out at sea like a mountain range cast adrift from the mainland.

Up a little farther, the trail widens to road width, and you can look can down upon Deer Canyon trail camp nestled in a grove of sycamores in the shallow canyon to your left. Still farther up the ridgeline, a gate across the road marks the boundary between the state park and the Laguna Coast Wilderness Park. Shy of this gate, however, you pick up the narrow Fenceline Trail on the right leading southeast toward El Moro Canyon, parallel to the boundary fence. After 0.4 mile on this trail, you hook up with a road coming in from the left. Keep straight momentarily, and just ahead turn left at the next junction. This puts you on the more scenic "Elevator Trail" east-side descent into upper El Moro Canyon, rather than the less scenic west-side descent called Slow 'N Easy Trail.

A steep (average 20 percent for 0.3 mile) grade follows, the bane of mountain bikers traveling either up or down, and hikers too. But afterward you can let

gravity repay you in a gentle way as you make a much more gradual descent along the bottom of El Moro Canyon.

Upper El Moro Canyon is far and away the most beautiful attraction in the park's backcountry. You stroll past thickets of willow, toyon, elderberry, and sycamore, all brightly illuminated by the sun; then you suddenly plunge into cool, dark, cathedral-like recesses overhung by the massive limbs of live oaks. In one such recess, several shallow caves, adorned with ferns at their entrances, pock a sandstone outcrop next to the road. Prior to the establishment of the California missions, coast-dwelling Indians gathered acorns, seeds, and wild berries in this canyon. These foods, coupled with the abundant marine life nearby, provided a balanced and healthy diet.

Continue down El Moro Canyon until you approach the trailer park (future campground) near the canyon's mouth. Make a right turn there and return to the visitor center.

El Moro Canyon, Crystal Cove State Park

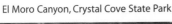

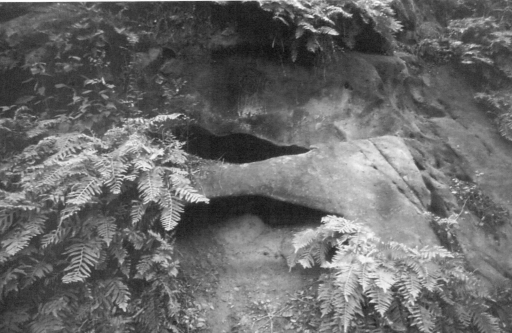

[TRIP 5] Deer Canyon Loop

Distance	7.1 miles, Loop
Hiking Time	4 hours
Elevation Gain/Loss	1300'/1300'
Difficulty	Moderately strenuous
Trail Use	Suitable for mountain biking, suitable for backpacking
Best Times	October through May
Agency	CCSP
Optional Map	USGS 7.5-min *Laguna Beach*
Notes	Marked trails/obvious routes, easy terrain

DIRECTIONS Crystal Cove State Park's visitor center and backcountry trailhead is located just east of Pacific Coast Highway, 2 miles north of Laguna Beach and 3 miles south of Corona del Mar. The entrance driveway is well marked, and a traffic light has been installed here for safety.

The Deer Canyon loop route along the west edge of Crystal Cove's backcountry sector explores the park's higher ridges and valleys. Since there's little shade along the way, and views are the primary attraction, the hike is by far most rewarding on clear, cool winter or early spring day. Backpackers have the option of staying overnight at Deer Canyon's trail camp, near the halfway point of the loop.

You begin hiking from the visitor center on No Dogs Road, with a no-nonsense ascent and an ever-widening view of El Moro Canyon below. That view is especially intriguing when the canyon bottom is filled with fog, as it often may be on late fall and winter mornings. Stay left at the next two junctions (Poles Road and West Cut-Across) and continue making your way north along the undulating ridgetop road called No Name Ridge Road. A vast area of new luxury homes comes into view on the left, completely contrasting with the open, protected lands of the state park on the right.

At 2.4 miles, No Name Ridge Road passes into Laguna Coast Wilderness Park

land. Before the gate, look for the narrow, rutty "Ticketron" trail branching right. Ticketron makes a radical drop (at least for mountain-bike riders) toward the floor of shallow Deer Canyon, then settles into an easy grade as it approaches the trail camp, which features a picnic bench, a composting toilet, and sites to pitch a tent down near a scraggly line of live oaks and sycamores.

Beyond the campground a short, steep climb leads to Redtail Ridge Trail, which is a fire road to the left (north) and a narrower trail to the right (south). Head south, following the top of the rounded ridge, and pass over an 844-foot knoll with a commanding ocean view. Then make a sharp descent to an old roadbed (Rattlesnake Trail) which continues downhill more moderately. You curl around Deer Canyon's small stream and meet West Cut-Across at a total of 5.1 miles.

For the remaining 2 miles, descend West Cut-Across to El Moro Canyon, follow the El Moro Canyon Trail downhill to the trailer park (future campground), and return to the visitor center on the 0.4 mile trail link on the right.

Chapter 4

Beaches and Bays:
Laguna Coast

The quintessentially coastal town of Laguna Beach blankets pillowy hills that rise abruptly from the sea to an elevation of nearly 1000 feet. Many of its finest houses cling precipitously to ledges cut into the steep slopes. Other houses seemingly defy gravity by resting upon cantilevered platforms or spidery networks of steel poles. There is an almost universal striving to capture a piece of the view, which without a doubt encompasses one of California's most dramatic stretches of coastline.

Laguna Beach residents have faced periodic disasters ranging from the loss of hundreds of homes in the Laguna Beach fire of 1993 to lesser catastrophes such as a landslide on a waterlogged slope that destroyed or destabilized dozens of hillside homes in early 2005. Many residents have rebuilt their homes after such incidents of misfortune.

Laguna residents have also been fiercely protective of the natural environment around their coastal town. In the 1980s and 90s they spearheaded a campaign to protect thousands of acres of land in and around Laguna Canyon slated for development. Those efforts reached a dramatic crescendo in 1989 when more than 8000 people marched down the road through Laguna Canyon protesting the Irvine Company's plan for a huge housing development there. In what many regard as a win-win outcome, the Irvine Company was allowed to proceed with massive urban development elsewhere, and large parcels of land such as the Laguna Coast Wilderness Park were created at the same time with the help of grants, donations, and park bond funds. Efforts continue to flesh out remaining parcels of potential parkland

Prickly pear cactus

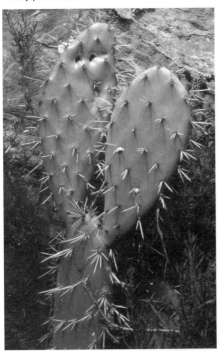

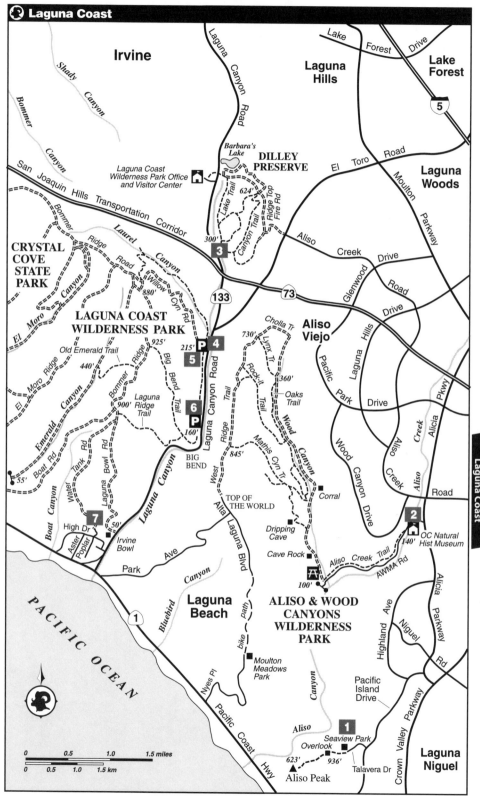

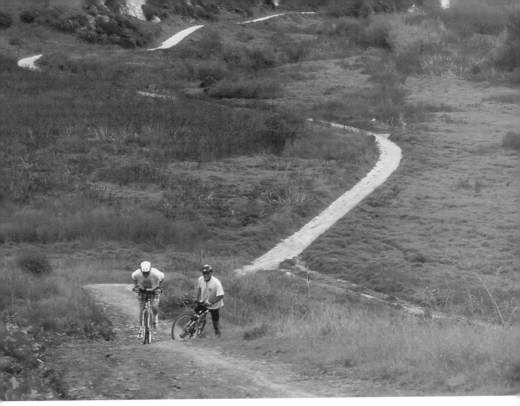

Mathis Canyon Trail

in the Laguna coast area. Similar cooper-
ative ventures are taking place farther
north involving Irvine Company lands in
the foothills of the Santa Ana Mountains.

Inland from Laguna Canyon and
Laguna Coast Wilderness Park, an older
park, the Aliso and Wood Canyons
Wilderness Park dedicated in 1979,
spreads across public utility lands and
other formerly private properties. The
park became an instant hit with all sorts
of self-propelled travelers when it
opened, though mountain-biking use
predominates there now.

Collectively, the contiguous open
spaces and parklands surrounding
Laguna Beach, including Crystal Cove
State Park, total nearly 20,000 acres. The
following seven hiking routes in Aliso
and Wood Canyons Regional Park and
Laguna Coast Wilderness Park will take
you to some of the finest overlooks along
the California coast and guide you into
many a quiet canyon recess.

TRIP 1 Seaview Park Overlook

Distance	0.5 mile or more, Out-and-back
Hiking Time	½ hour
Difficulty	Easy
Trail Use	Good for kids
Best Times	All year
Agency	AWCWP
Optional Map	USGS 7.5-min *San Juan Capistrano*
Notes	Marked trails/obvious routes, easy terrain

DIRECTIONS Follow Pacific Island Drive either 1.6 miles north from Crown Valley Parkway or 1.2 miles south from Alicia Parkway to reach Talavera Drive. Follow Talavera 0.3 mile west to its end at Seaview Park.

Starting from Seaview Park in the city of Laguna Niguel, this brief walk will take you past several interpretive panels annotating the common species of coastal vegetation found throughout coastal Southern California. The path leads to a concrete platform offering a jaw-dropping view of the hills of Laguna Beach spilling down to the ocean. If you live in Orange County, this somewhat obscure overlook is a good spot to keep in mind when entertaining out-of-town relatives or friends.

You start at the end of Talavera Drive, off Pacific Island Drive, 1.6 miles north of Crown Valley Parkway. On some maps, the starting point is identified as Niguel Hill (936′). Start walking at the west end of the grassy strip running along the brink of Aliso Canyon. Follow a wide, ridge-running path going west. Notice the differences between the types of vegetation growing on the two sides of the path. Dense chaparral clings to the steep, north-facing slope to the right, which drops a sheer 800 feet to Aliso Creek. A sparser assemblage of mostly coastal-sage-scrub plants lies exposed to the sun's harshest rays on the left, south-facing, side of the path.

Only a few minutes walk takes you to the concrete platform. Most casual hikers will likely want to turn back there. Beyond the platform, a narrower trail continues: it pitches sharply downward, skirts a residential street, and then rises a little to reach Aliso Peak (Aliso Summit). From there the ocean shore lies just 0.4 mile away—600 feet below.

Laguna Coast

Cavernous sandstone

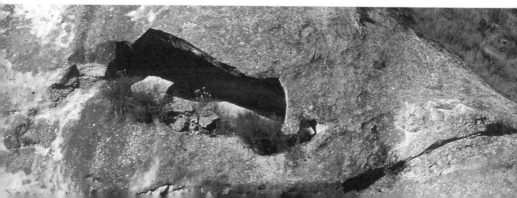

TRIP 2 Aliso and Wood Canyons Loop

Distance	10.0 miles, Loop
Hiking Time	5 hours
Elevation Gain/Loss	950'/950'
Difficulty	Moderately strenuous
Trail Use	Suitable for mountain biking
Best Times	November through June
Agency	AWCWP
Optional Map	USGS 7.5-min *San Juan Capistrano, Laguna Beach*
Notes	Marked trails/obvious routes, easy terrain

DIRECTIONS Aliso/Wood Canyon's primary trailhead is located opposite Laguna Niguel Regional Park and adjacent to the Orange County Natural History Museum on Alicia Parkway, 0.2 mile south of Aliso Creek Road in Laguna Niguel.

Aliso and Wood Canyons Wilderness Park consists of over 4200 acres of shallow canyons, sandstone rock formations, narrow strips of oak and riparian woodland, and hillsides draped with aromatic sage-scrub vegetation. Subdivisions and subdivisions-in-the-making press in along the park's long, narrow boundary, which is perforated by many neighborhood access points.

This trip takes you on a grand, looping tour of the Wood Canyon section of the park. The park's multiuse trails accommodate all sorts of self-propelled travelers. You will unavoidably encounter passing mountain bikes, though our route does try to avoid the trails most favored by mountain bikers. I recommend that you try to explore the park during the gorgeous "green" months of February through April. During the summer, the midday hours are uncomfortably warm, though the early morning and pre-sunset periods are often fairly cool. The park is open daily, 7 A.M. to sunset.

The sole trail departing the parking lot takes you subtly downhill along the wide floodplain of Aliso Canyon. This first part is, frankly, unexciting. You follow the shoulder of the AWMA access road for about 0.7 mile, then diverge on a trail that stays within a short distance of the road. The glimpses you get of sandstone outcrops on hillsides to the north are intriguing. This sandstone was derived from layers of sand deposited in an offshore environment some 15 million years ago. Soon you will see a lot more of this sandstone at close range.

At 1.4 miles you arrive at a major junction, with restrooms and benches, where the two canyons—Aliso and Wood—join. Head north on Wood Canyon Trail (the dirt road up Wood Canyon) and you soon spy, on the left, Cave Rock, a series of "wind caves" pocking a sandstone ledge. When weak sedimentary rock such as this is exposed to air and dripping water, the effects of chemical weathering loosen the mineral grains that are cemented together in the rock. Winds then scour out hollows such as you see here.

Continue north on the Wood Canyon Trail until, at 2.2 miles, you find and follow the side trail on the left leading to Dripping Cave. This impressive overhang, tucked into a narrow ravine, was the supposed hideout of 19th century stagecoach and livestock thieves. Holes bored into the cave's walls once held pegs used to hang supplies, and the black color of the cave's ceiling is evidence of past campfires. Ferns cling to the ledge above the cave, nourished by dripping water during much of the year.

Retrace your steps for a few paces and veer left on the narrow trail going northwest. You contour across a steep hillside, pass some elaborately sculpted sandstone formations on the far side of a ravine, and drop precariously onto the flat floor of

Dripping Cave

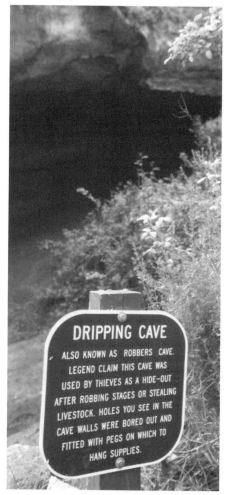

DRIPPING CAVE

ALSO KNOWN AS ROBBERS CAVE. LEGEND CLAIM THIS CAVE WAS USED BY THIEVES AS A HIDE-OUT AFTER ROBBING STAGES OR STEALING LIVESTOCK. HOLES YOU SEE IN THE CAVE WALLS WERE BORED OUT AND FITTED WITH PEGS ON WHICH TO HANG SUPPLIES.

shallow Mathis Canyon. Turn left on the Mathis Canyon Trail and stay right at the next split. A 500-foot, no-nonsense climb atop a narrow ridge ensues. This may be eased by the pauses you take to admire the ever-widening views of Wood Canyon—an island of green or gold amid an endless suburban tapestry spreading inland. Hawks, ravens, and vultures patrol the air space around you, gliding by at close range or spiraling upward on thermals.

At 3.8 miles, the sweaty ascent ends as you reach the West Ridge Trail, a wide, graded fire road coming down from the "Top of the World" neighborhood in the city of Laguna Beach. Turn right (north) and enjoy fine views of the sharp gash of Laguna Canyon to the left and the more gentle watershed of Wood Canyon on the right. At 5.2 miles, find and follow the narrow Lynx Trail on the right (very steep in a couple of spots) down a ridge and into upper Wood Canyon. On this trail the viewshed is pristine—no sign of anything other than precipitous hillsides clothed in dense chaparral and live oaks. The breeze blowing up the canyon often bears the scent of marine air tinged with sage.

At the bottom of the Lynx Trail, turn right on the Wood Canyon Trail. Close ahead, veer right on the Oaks Trail, a parallel trail down the canyon for hiking-only traffic (if you are on a mountain bike, stay on Wood Canyon Trail). Following a narrow strip of oak woodland along the Oaks Trail, and later the Coyote Run Trail, you reach—after nearly 2 miles of travel in shady Wood Canyon—Mathis Canyon Trail. Veer left to cross Wood Canyon's tiny creek and to hook up with the Wood Canyon Trail again. Continue south to the Aliso-Wood canyon confluence, and from there return to the Alicia Parkway trailhead the way you came.

Laguna Coast

TRIP 3 Dilley Preserve

Distance	2.9 miles, Loop
Hiking Time	1½ hours
Elevation Gain/Loss	350'/350'
Difficulty	Moderate
Trail Use	Good for kids
Best Times	All year
Agency	LCWP
Optional Map	USGS 7.5-min *Laguna Beach*
Notes	Marked trails/obvious routes, easy terrain

DIRECTIONS Park at the Dilley Preserve staging area on the east side of Laguna Canyon Road, 4 miles south of Interstate 405, and just north of the Highway 73 toll-road offramps.

The James Dilley Greenbelt Preserve, a unit within the Laguna Coast Wilderness Park, dates back to a landmark purchase by the city of Laguna Beach in 1978. Environmentalist James Dilley helped champion the concept of "greenbelts," or parcels of open space between cityscapes, back in that era.

The trail system in the preserve is pieced together out of former bulldozed roads and current utility roads. The 2.9-mile loop described here covers the best trails and touches upon the best sights the preserve has to offer. The first stretch (Canyon Trail) doubles as a portion of the 1.8-mile long Bea Whittlesly Loop self-guiding nature trail, which features posts keyed to a brochure available at the trailhead.

From the Dilley staging area, head east across a field of sage and buckwheat on the Canyon Trail, which at first gains elevation gradually and stays near the bottom of small canyon dotted with gorgeous specimens of coast live oak and California sycamore. At about 0.7 mile the trail begins a steeper ascent, curling upward through a patch of prickly-pear cactus (look or listen for cactus wrens).

At 1.0 mile, you arrive on top of a buried water reservoir on a 624-foot knoll. Take a look around. The Leisure World development lies to the east, the open spaces of the Laguna Coast Wilderness Park sprawl to the south and west, and the winter-snowcapped summit of Mount San Antonio floats above the often-hazy urban landscape in the north.

Next, slip down the slope east of the reservoir to reach a maintained fire road following the ridge top. You'll want to head north—not on the gravel road that descends smoothly to the north and east, but rather on the somewhat rougher "Edison" road on the right that stays more or less underneath the high-voltage power lines. That route takes you down to and then right along the shoreline of beautiful Barbara's Lake, the larger of two small lakes that constitute Orange County's only naturally formed inland bodies of water. The lakes are geologically described as small sag ponds, located where the ground has subsided due to movements along a fault. Since Barbara's Lake is shallow and its drainage area is small, it is believed that artesian springs on the lake bottom help keep it full no

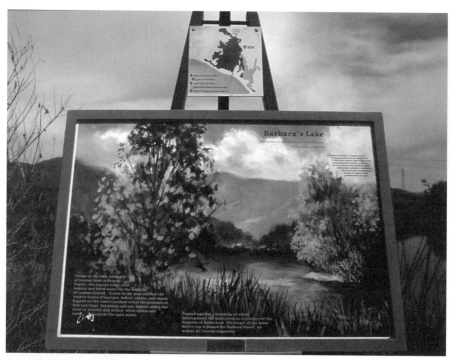

Painterly exhibit at Barbara's Lake

matter what the season. Barbara's Lake actually "expanded" in 2005 following the realignment and widening of Laguna Canyon Road. The old roadbed, which formerly divided Barbara's Lake from Bubbles Pond, has been obliterated, and the two bodies of water have joined together. Another lake, a seasonal body of water called Lake 1, lies about ½ mile north along Laguna Canyon Road.

At Barbara's Lake and elsewhere in the Laguna Coast Wilderness Park, you will find large plaques with original plein-air paintings by local artists. Ultraviolet-resistant coatings on the paintings have kept them from fading much over a number of years.

From the gravel road at the south end of Barbara's Lake, you can make a side trip under Laguna Canyon Road's arched overpasses to reach the James and Rosemary Nix Nature Center on the far side (slated for completion in 2006 or 2007). What are the strange cavities on the undersides of those overpasses? They are entrances into the hollow interiors of the concrete structures for use by bats and swallows.

Exclusive of the side trip under the overpasses, our designated 2.9-mile route goes south from the gravel road on nearly a bee-line course back to the starting point of the hike.

[Note: As of this writing, the Dilley preserve was closed and inaccessible due to Caltrans construction. The Laguna Canyon Road realignment and the restoration and reopening of the preserve will likely take place in 2006.]

TRIP 4 Laurel Canyon Loop

Distance	3.5 miles, Loop
Hiking Time	2 hours
Elevation Gain/Loss	700'/700'
Difficulty	Moderate
Trail Use	Good for kids
Best Times	All year
Agency	LCWP
Optional Map	USGS 7.5-min *Laguna Beach*
Notes	Marked trails/obvious routes, easy terrain

DIRECTIONS Park at Laguna Coast Wilderness Park's Willow Canyon staging area on the west side of Laguna Canyon Road, 3 miles north of Laguna Beach. This point is 5 miles south of Interstate 405, 0.7 mile south of the Highway 73 toll road, and 0.2 mile south of the El Toro Road/Laguna Canyon Road intersection.

The best single hike within the Laguna Coast Wilderness Park is surely the secluded Laguna Canyon loop. Though it lies close to the San Joaquin Hills Transportation Corridor tollway, that roadway and much associated urban development is hidden from both sight and sound along most of the route.

Volunteers frequently staff a booth at the Willow Canyon staging area, offering tips about the logistics of hiking in the park as well as natural history. Follow the fire road beyond—Willow Canyon Road, which gains nearly 600 feet of elevation in the next 1.5 miles. Springtime wildflowers bloom in profusion along this stretch, which cuts along east and north-facing slopes smothered in thick chaparral vegetation.

At 1.5 miles, turn right on the first intersecting pathway. Traverse a grassy meadow, and then follow the trail as it plunges down through more dense growths of chaparral toward the narrow bottom of Laurel Canyon. The deeper you go, the more you gain a sense of seclusion. Once you arrive in the canyon bottom (2.0 miles), don't miss the turn

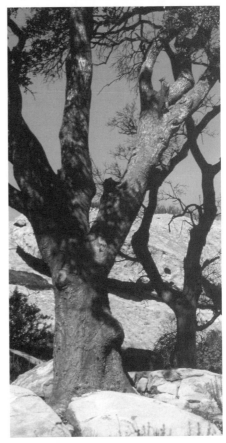

Singed oaks along Laurel Canyon Trail

onto the narrow trail that branches right and goes down (not up) the canyon.

Graced with gorgeous oaks and sycamores (and copious growths of poison oak), Laurel Canyon is still recovering from the extremely hot and fast-moving Laguna Beach fire of October 1993. Nearly all of the vegetation you see here is no stranger to periodic fires. Centuries ago, coastal Southern California landscapes such as this were visited by fire every decade or so.

At 2.4 miles, you pass near the lip of a dramatic dropoff—a seasonal waterfall nearly 100 feet high. During the extraordinarily wet winter of 2005, hikers beheld a spectacular sight of plunging water, but most years this declivity sports only a modest trickle.

Past the lip of the falls, you swing to the left side of the canyon bottom, and descend along a dry, south-facing slope. By 3.0 miles you emerge in a grassy meadow, which is either green, golden, or transitional in color, depending on the season. Cavernous sandstone outcrops dot the meadow on the left and the slope on the right. The shapes of some suggest grotesque skulls and other figures. The path through the meadow soon flanks busy Laguna Canyon Road, and you arrive back at your parked car.

TRIP 5 Emerald Canyon

Distance	8.4 miles round trip (to falls in Emerald Canyon), Out-and-back
Hiking Time	4 hours (round trip)
Elevation Gain/Loss	1400'/1400'
Difficulty	Moderately strenuous
Trail Use	Suitable for mountain biking
Best Times	November through May
Agency	LCWP
Optional Map	USGS 7.5-min *Laguna Beach*
Notes	Marked trails/obvious routes, easy terrain

DIRECTIONS Park at Laguna Coast Wilderness Park's Willow Canyon staging area on the west side of Laguna Canyon Road, 3 miles north of Laguna Beach. This point is 5 miles south of Interstate 405, 0.7 mile south of the Highway 73 toll road, and 0.2 mile south of the El Toro Road/Laguna Canyon Road intersection.

Equally as beautiful as El Moro Canyon in neighboring Crystal Cove State Park, Emerald Canyon receives much less visitation. This is due to the "landlocked" status of its lower end. Access to the canyon is from above only. Entry into the lower end of the canyon by way of Laguna Beach's city streets is blocked by a formidable fence.

Both hikers and mountain bikers can follow the route as described here. Hikers and gonzo mountain bikers, either on the way out or the way back if they choose, can also follow a somewhat longer variant of the route by utilizing the single-track, often overgrown Old Emerald Trail.

Follow Willow Canyon Road 1.5 miles to the Laurel Canyon turnoff, but stay straight (south) and climb 0.1 mile to an intersection with Bommer Ridge Road. Turn right, proceed 0.1 mile to a dip in the road, and turn left onto Emerald Canyon Road. That "road"—essentially a wide trail—descends along the top of ridge for a mile, through growths of sage, encelia, and monkeyflowers blooming in shades from orange to yellow.

After a mile on the descending ridge, you arrive on the canyon bottom, at a place where the narrow Old Emerald Trail obscurely branches left. The next 1.5 miles of travel down-canyon is along a more moderate grade, and the scenery is simply gorgeous. Gnarled oaks and sycamores—survivors of repeated firestorms—line the trail, and dense willow growth flanks the canyon's seasonal stream. Take care not to brush against the luxuriant growths of poison oak on both sides of the trail. About halfway down this easy stretch, note the spacious cave pocking a large sandstone outcrop on the left, across the canyon bottom.

At 4.2 miles from the start, you arrive at a place where the trail curls sharply downward and a 20-foot-high waterfall lies to the right. This waterfall is more like a "dry fall" in most years, and comes alive only with sustained heavy rains. This is a good spot to take a break, and afterward return the way you came. The remaining half mile down to and back from the secure fence at the edge of Laguna Beach is worth exploring only if you have energy to spare.

Sandstone caves, Emerald Canyon

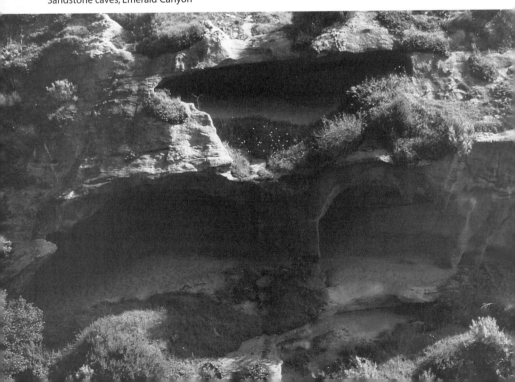

TRIP 6 Big Bend Loop

Distance	4.5 miles, Loop
Hiking Time	3 hours
Elevation Gain/Loss	1100'/1100'
Difficulty	Moderate
Best Times	November through May
Agency	LCWP
Optional Map	USGS 7.5-min *Laguna Beach*
Notes	Marked trails/obvious routes, moderate terrain

DIRECTIONS Park at Laguna Coast Wilderness Park's Big Bend parking lot on the west side of Laguna Canyon Road, 2 miles north of Laguna Beach and 2 miles south of the Highway 73 toll road.

Both the beginning part on Big Bend Trail and the ending part on Laguna Ridge Trail will test the mettle of any hiker, due to a combination of steepness and roughness. Although mountain bikes are technically allowed on the route, much of that effort would go into slinging the bike over one's shoulder and slip-sliding down the steepest grades. You might as well walk!

The low-growing coastal sage-scrub and grassland vegetation on the slopes and ridges hereabouts does little to block views of the ocean, hills, and distant mountains. This is a hike best taken, then, whenever the air is beautifully transparent.

From the Big Bend staging area, head south and start climbing immediately on the Big Bend Trail. At 0.2 mile, just as you cross under some power lines, note the obscure path to the left. You will arrive at this spot again near the end of the hike.

The Big Bend Trail takes you ever upward along a ridgeline on a course absolutely committed to gaining elevation as quickly as possible. A couple of flat stretches along the way, though, allow you to catch your breath and look around. Before long, cars and buildings in

Laguna Canyon below begin to look toy-like. Scallop fossils can be spotted lying near your passing feet if your eyes are glued to the ground.

At 1.6 miles you come to an intersection with the wide Bommer Ridge Road. Turn left and proceed south on a gently falling, then gently rising course to the intersection of Boat Canyon Road on the right (2.7 miles from the start). On the left, just past Boat Canyon Road but before the next intersecting road on the right, a narrow track goes briefly up a 912-foot knoll, then suddenly and precipitously plunges down. This is the Laguna Ridge Trail that will take you back down to Laguna Canyon.

Rough and worn deeply into the sandstone bedrock, the Laguna Ridge Trail approaches a 40 percent grade in a couple of spots. It, too, sticks to a plunging ridgeline. Nearing the bottom of that plunge, the trail veers left (east), almost reaching the pavement of Laguna Canyon Road (3.6 miles). The final mile or so of trail goes up and down a couple of times, staying parallel to but decently clear of the busy roadway. At 4.3 miles you meet Big Bend Trail, which leads 0.2 mile down to the starting point.

Laguna Coast

TRIP 7 Laguna Bowl Loop

Distance	3.6 miles, Loop
Hiking Time	2 hours
Elevation Gain/Loss	950'/950'
Difficulty	Moderate
Trail Use	Suitable for mountain biking
Best Times	All year
Agency	LCWP
Optional Map	USGS 7.5-min *Laguna Beach*
Notes	Marked trails/obvious routes, easy terrain

DIRECTIONS Follow Aster Street north from Pacific Coast Highway in Laguna Beach. Continue 0.3 mile to High Drive; go right one block, and turn left on Poplar Street. Follow Poplar to its end and park on the street.

On many a fall or winter morning, a damp, opaque layer of air a few hundred feet deep lies over the low-lying Southern California coast. By 9 or 10 in the morning, the sun usually "burns" through this marine-layer fog, ushering in a fine day of mild sunshine. Sleepy-eyed hikers never know what they're missing unless they seize the moment and get an early start on any coastal hiking route, such as this one, that pokes above the cloud layer.

Squeeze through a gate at the east end of Poplar Street and start up a very steep paved road. After 0.1 mile, the paved road enters a fenced water-tank and antenna facility, but a steep bypass trail skirts the fenced area on the right and keeps climbing. Soon that bypass joins a dirt road-bed, the Water Tank Road. You continue climbing, but more moderately. At about 0.4 mile and 550 feet of elevation, you enter Laguna Coast Wilderness Park property. The early-morning boundary between fog and clear air often lies at about this level. If that is the case when you're there, then the next couple of miles will be an absolute delight.

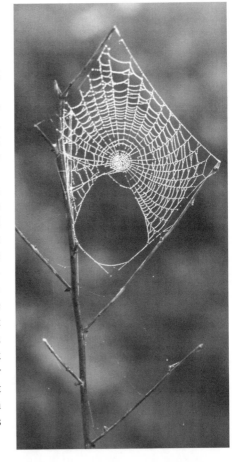

Spider web

Right at the boundary between clear air and cloud, look westward (opposite the rising sun) and you may see the upper arc of a colorless rainbow (the so-called white rainbow) that results from sunlight refracting through water droplets much smaller than those of falling rain. Another remarkable spectacle, called the "glory" or "Specter of the Brocken," is visible whenever you can manage to cast the shadow of your own body onto a bank of fog. The ghostly specter is that of concentric rings of colored light at the spot exactly 180 degrees away from the sun. The right conditions and optical geometry exists during the first hour or so after sunrise.

At 1.5 miles you arrive at the junction of Bommer Ridge Road (to the left) and Laguna Bowl Road (to the right). Turn right, head south along the top of the ridgeline, and enjoy vistas of the blue ocean ahead, or of tendrils of fog below, depending on the atmospheric conditions. At 2.2 miles the road forks; take the right branch, staying on Laguna Bowl Road. Soon afterward you commence a quick, steep descent that takes you past the fenced Irvine Bowl outdoor amphitheater and down to Laguna Canyon Road.

To complete the loop you must follow city streets. Turn right, follow the sidewalk of Laguna Canyon Road for 0.25 mile, turn right on Acacia Drive, and immediately go right on High Drive. Follow High Drive for 0.25 mile, and turn right on Poplar Street to return to your car.

Laguna Coast

Chapter 5

Beaches and Bays:
South Coast

L ife seems to pass a little more slowly
along Orange County's southernmost
stretch of coastline. Somewhat removed
from the snarling traffic and the crush of
people upcoast, the narrow beaches and
eroded cliffs are quite in tune with the
rhythm of the surf and the tides. While
Dana Point, Capistrano Beach, and San
Clemente continue to fill up with elegant
houses and condominium complexes
spilling over the coastal bluffs and
foothills, these communities still boast
many miles of tranquil beach. Away from
the main focal points of activity, you can
still enjoy a warm evening's stroll on the
sand with nothing but shorebirds as companions.

In this section, I'll elaborate on two
fine coastal walks in south Orange
County, plus a third (San Onofre State
Beach) just over the line in San Diego
County. I've included the latter because it
is readily accessible to Orange Countians.

Replica of the *Pilgrim*

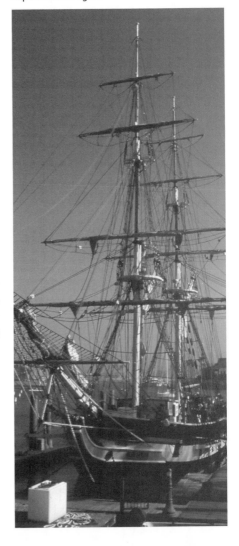

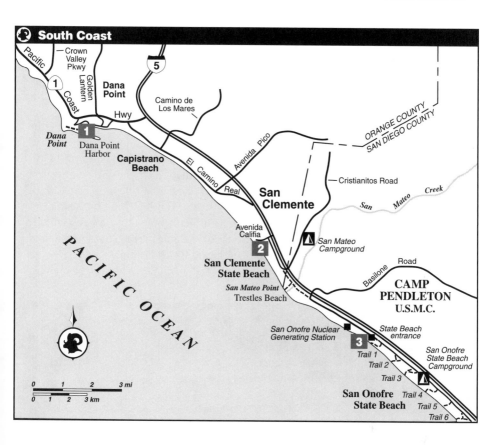

South Coast

Crown Valley Pkwy
Golden Lantern
Dana Point
1
Pacific Coast Hwy
5
Camino de Los Mares
ORANGE COUNTY
SAN DIEGO COUNTY
Dana Point
1
Dana Point Harbor
Capistrano Beach
El Camino Real
Avenida Pico
Cristianitos Road
San Mateo Creek
San Clemente
Avenida Califia
2
San Mateo Campground
San Clemente State Beach
San Mateo Point Trestles Beach
Basilone Road
CAMP PENDLETON U.S.M.C.
San Onofre Nuclear Generating Station
State Beach entrance
3
San Onofre State Beach Campground
Trail 1
Trail 2
Trail 3
San Onofre State Beach
Trail 4
Trail 5
Trail 6

PACIFIC OCEAN

0   1   2   3 mi
0   1   2   3 km

TRIP 1 Dana Point Headlands

Distance	1.4 miles round trip, Out-and-back
Hiking Time	1 hour (round trip)
Difficulty	Easy
Trail Use	Good for kids
Best Times	Low tide; October through March
Agency	OIDP
Optional Map	USGS 7.5-min *Dana Point*
Notes	Marked trails/obvious routes, moderate terrain

DIRECTIONS From Pacific Coast Highway, just west of Dana Point's "downtown," turn south on Street of the Green Lantern. Drive 2 blocks south to Cove Road and turn left. Cove Road descends to Dana Point Harbor Drive and Dana Cove Park, where the beach walk begins.

The sea cliffs at Dana Point are revered by historians as the site where Spanish vaqueros threw hides over the cliffs and down to waiting ships as described in Richard Henry Dana's *Two Years Before the Mast*. Today, the sheer cliffs remain, but much of coastline below is occupied by the 2500-slip Dana Point Marina. Just west of that marina, though, you'll find a fine wild stretch of rocky beach and dramatic headland, a little piece of Old California that can be fully explored during low tides.

Just beyond the starting point, the Dana Cove Park parking lot, you'll find a replica of the *Pilgrim*, the sailing ship that author Dana sailed on during the early 1800s, and the Ocean Institute museum. Beyond the museum, descend a stairway to the beach and (tide permitting) pick your way westward over storm tossed boulders and under the looming cliffs toward the rocky headland of Dana Point itself. The mostly metamorphic rocks underfoot, having a variety of colors and textures, have eroded out of the conglomerate cliffs.

There's a sea cave at the end of the walkable section (0.7 mile from the parking lot), and plenty of small sea stacks just offshore that catch the incoming waves and breakers. The tidepools here are of fair quality. Travel beyond the sea cave is more difficult, but with a low enough tide you may be able to reach the smooth sand of Strand Beach beyond.

Sea cave at Dana Point

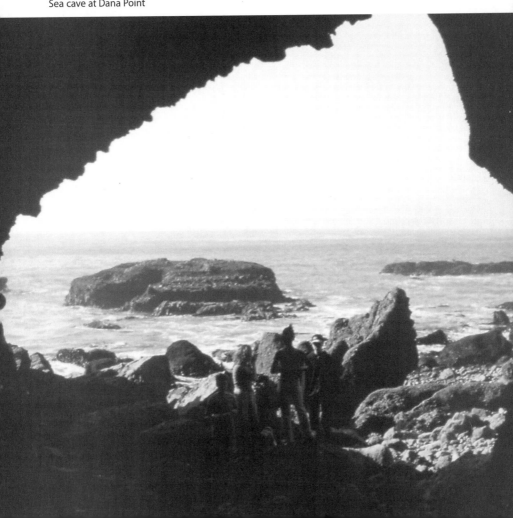

TRIP 2 San Clemente State Beach

Distance	3 miles, Loop
Hiking Time	1½ hours
Elevation Gain/Loss	150'/150'
Difficulty	Easy
Trail Use	Good for kids
Best Times	All year
Agency	SCSB
Optional Map	USGS 7.5-min *San Clemente*
Notes	Marked trails/obvious routes, easy terrain

DIRECTIONS From southbound Interstate 5, exit at Avenida Calafia in San Clemente and drive west ¼ mile to the San Clemente State Beach entrance.

From Dana Point to San Mateo Point, a long, gently curving stretch of sand and surf beckons surfers, swimmers, sunbathers, and strollers. In the north half, both the old coast highway and the tracks of the Santa Fe Railroad follow the beach. South into San Clemente, the highway turns inland, while the tracks, chiseled along the base of tan-colored cliffs, continue near the tideline.

South of San Clemente State Beach, the coastline is scenic and isolated, and it receives few visitors—good reasons why ex-President Richard Nixon located his "Western White House" here. Only the sudden thunder of a passing train, every half-hour or so, disturbs the beachgoer's reverie of curling breakers, shifting sands, and salt-laden breezes.

On the loop route described here you begin by walking on the sand, but return via an inland route that skirts the mouth of San Mateo Creek.

From the day-use area of San Clemente State Beach, descend to the sand on either of the two trails that drop 120 feet through gaps in the cliff wall. The cliffs, consisting of marine deposits about 15 million years old, form the blunt edge of the marine terrace on which much of the city of San Clemente rests. Today, the forces of erosion, including the not-insignificant pitter-patter of countless bare feet down the paths and the chiseling of inscriptions in the rock, help to loosen sand grains and hasten their return to the sea.

Cross the tracks through an underpass and head south along the beach onto a posted stretch overlooked by a row of modern homes. Although the upper beach is private here, California law protects public use and passage below the mean-high-tide line.

Tall palms and cypress trees on the left conceal most of the former Western White House, but a round structure—the "Card Room," where Nixon and Dwight Eisenhower used to enjoy card games—is perched on the cliff edge.

The cliffs peter out at San Mateo Point, where Orange County ends and San Diego County begins. In the water gap just ahead lies the marshy mouth of San Mateo Creek. On the right is Trestles Beach (part of San Onofre State Beach), a favorite of surfers. Ahead a little and back of the white sand lies a shallow, cattail-fringed pond where San Mateo Creek comes to an inglorious end after winding more than 20 miles from the southern Santa Ana and Santa Margarita mountains. Only during wet periods does the flow of water breach the sand to reach the ocean. This a good place to watch migratory birds, especially in winter.

Head inland now by crossing under the low railroad trestle that gave the beach its name. Pick up a paved service road/bike path, often clogged with surfers portaging their boards. After 0.3 mile, you'll reach the main bicycle path paralleling Interstate 5 through Camp Pendleton. Turn left (north) here and after 0.2 mile you'll come up to Avenida del Presidente, the west frontage road of I-5. Follow Avenida del Presidente another 0.8 mile north to Avenida San Luis Rey, where a pedestrian pass-through on the left leads into the fenced San Clemente State Beach campground.

TRIP 3 San Onofre State Beach

Distance	1 to 6 miles
Difficulty	Easy to moderate
Trail Use	Good for kids
Best Times	All year
Agency	SOSB
Optional Map	USGS 7.5-min *San Onofre Bluff*
Notes	Marked trails/obvious routes, easy terrain

DIRECTIONS Exit Interstate 5 at Basilone Road in Camp Pendleton, just south of San Clemente. Turn west and follow the westside frontage road (Old Highway 101) for 3 miles to the main San Onofre State Beach entrance.

San Onofre State Beach is perhaps best known as a busy camping spot midway between the Los Angeles and San Diego metropolitan areas. More than 300 campsites serve the needs of traveling motorists, touring bicyclists, and (rarely) backpackers headed up or down the coast.

The state beach includes three parcels of land leased from the Marine Corps, whose big Camp Pendleton base sprawls for 17 miles down the coast from San Clemente. A north coastal section extends from the Orange County line (Trestles Beach) to the San Onofre Nuclear Generating Station. The second, most heavily used section lies south of the power station, and consists of 3 miles of beach and ocean bluff just west of Interstate 5. The 300 or so campsites here occupy the roadbed of the former U.S. Highway 101, and all are impacted by traffic noise from freeway. A third parcel of state park territory lies inland along Cristianitos Road. It includes San Mateo Campground, a quiet and serene place to camp for now—until and unless the proposed Foothill Transporation Corridor freeway is extended this far south in the latter part of this decade.

It's worth taking at least a brief look at the sage-scrub vegetation on top of the bluffs. These are fairly dense and undisturbed stands, accented with taller shrubs like laurel sumac, lemonade berry, toyon, and tree tobacco. Red and sticky monkeyflower plants are here, producing a variety of colors during the spring bloom: red, orange, salmon pink, and yellow. The red variety is a great attractor of hummingbirds. Bladderpod, a familiar plant of California's deserts, also makes a home among the sage scrub here.

Several dirt roads or pathways, designated Trails 1 through 6, travel through ravines or breaks in the bluff wall to reach the white-sand beach below. There, the sounds and sights of civilization are gone, and you're left to explore a primeval stretch of coastline. Strolling along the water's edge, you may spot dolphins, sea lions, and harbor seals. My companions and I once watched a pair of dolphins cavorting in the surf less than 50 feet from the shore.

A secluded stretch of beach south of the southernmost trail, Trail 6, extending into Camp Pendelton receives de facto, though not officially sanctioned use by nudists.

In the northern reaches of the beach, north of Trail 1 and extending to as far as the nuclear power plant, the eroded cliff faces rising over the beach are especially interesting and photogenic. In color and form, some are reminiscent of the formations in Utah's Bryce Canyon National Park.

At a point 0.6 mile south of the power plant, note how the line of bold cliffs ends suddenly. Look upward through the vegetation to discover the Cristianitos Fault, a crack in the earth that extends some 25 miles inland. To the right (south) side of the fault's inclined surface you'll see the brownish Monterey shale, a fine-grained sedimentary rock deposited some 15 to 20 million years ago. To the left of the fault is the off-white San Mateo sandstone, laid down an estimated 5 million

Bluffs north of Trail 1

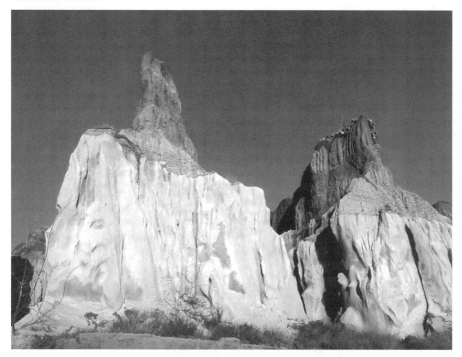

years ago. Above both of these formations lies a flat, continuous layer of boulders deposited in a marine environment about 120,000 years ago, and other land-laid deposits on top of the bouldery layer. The undisturbed nature of these upper layers has assured geologists that the Cristianitos Fault has been moribund for at least 120,000 years and therefore is almost certainly not a threat to the stability and safety of the nuclear power plant. Other faults, however, are known to exist several miles to the southwest. These offshore faults are thought to be extensions of faults exposed on land that are known to have been active in historic times.

You can spend as little as a half hour or as much as half a day exploring the 3+ miles of beachfront that lies below the bluffs. Remember that it is easier to walk this sandy stretch during low tide, taking advantage of the wet, hard-packed sand just above the reach of the surging waves.

Beach north of Trail 1

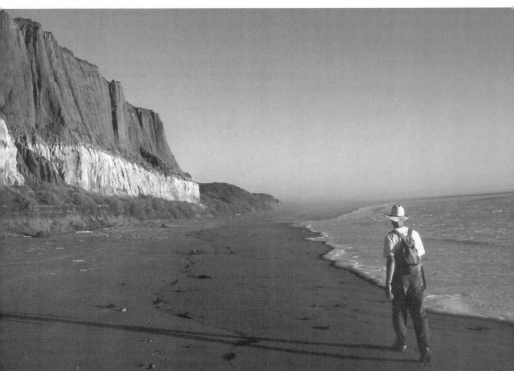

Chapter 6

Foothills:
Chino Hills

Seen from the air, the Chino Hills look like a rumpled bedsheet tossed near the northern brow of the higher Santa Ana Mountains. If they weren't cleanly separated from the Santa Anas by the broad trench of Santa Ana Canyon, these hills and their extensions to the north, the Puente Hills, would certainly be considered the northernmost expressions of the Peninsular Ranges.

Rapidly eroding, yet exhibiting a rather graceful, rounded topography, the Chino Hills consist of 5- to 15-million-year-old marine sedimentary rocks uplifted fairly recently by movements along the Whittier fault zone to the west and along lesser faults to the east. The maximum thickness of these sediments—called the Puente Formation—in the Chino Hills is 13,000 feet.

For the past two centuries the rolling, grassy swells and wooded ravines of the Chino Hills have been used for cattle and sheep grazing. Originally they were a part of lands assigned to Mission San Gabriel; later they were incorporated into various Spanish land grants or reserved as lands in the public domain. Private ranching interests acquired most of the land by the mid-20th Century. By the 1970s, however, ranching was in decline everywhere around Southern California and tract houses began popping up like mush-

rooms around the base of the hills. The setting aside of open space and parkland suddenly became an urgent priority.

In 1975 Orange County established the 124-acre Carbon Canyon Regional Park on the west edge of the Chino Hills. Following suit, the State of California in 1977 began a feasibility study for a large park in the Chino Hills. In 1981 the state acquired its first parcel, and by 1984 Chino Hills State Park was opened to the public. Today, after the expenditure of over $50 million, nearly 13,000 acres of state parkland stretch from Carbon Canyon Regional Park to the eastern edge of the Chino Hills in San Bernardino and Riverside counties. The park remains almost entirely undeveloped today, containing just one small drive-in campground, an equestrian staging area, and scattered picnic tables and privies. Future improvements may include several large-capacity drive-in campgrounds, and a half-dozen trail camps for overnight travelers.

Aside from its recreational potential, Chino Hills State Park contains important plant and wildlife habitats. About 10 percent of the park's land area is classified as southern oak woodland, a plant community that has been greatly affected by California's population explosion. Some of the best remaining stands of the California walnut, a tree whose native range is

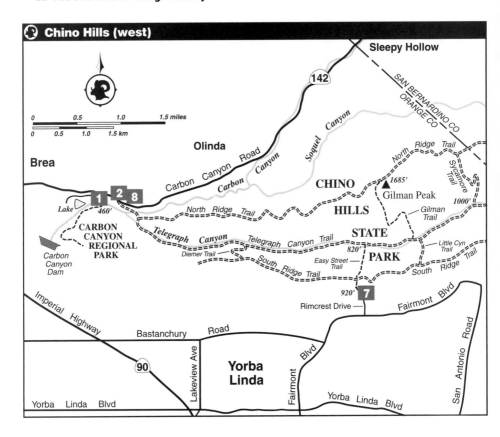

Chino Hills (west)

confined to the Los Angeles Basin and surrounding foothills, are found in the larger canyons of the park.

Wildlife includes mule deer, foxes, rabbits, coyotes, bobcats, badgers, mountain lions, and rattlesnakes. Several rare or endangered species of birds may visit the park, including the southern bald eagle, peregrine falcon, least Bell's vireo, California gnatcatcher, and the coastal cactus wren. From a biological perspective, the Chino Hills are regarded as a key link in a natural wildlife corridor stretching between the Whittier and Puente hills in the Los Angeles Basin to the Santa Ana Mountains in Orange and Riverside counties.

Chino Hills State Park is popular with hikers, equestrians, and especially mountain bicyclists, all of whom who enjoy the park's primitive character. Dirt roads and old cowpaths lace the open ridgelines and thread through the shady canyons. Some 60 miles of dirt roads and trails are open to mountain bikers as well as hikers and horse riders. Certain "single track" (narrower) trails may be closed to cyclists or equestrians. Trail signs and the allowed uses of the trails are now posted throughout the park, and an improved trail map available on entry into the park makes navigation relatively easy. The major trails and roads feature mile posts stating the distance (by way of the most direct route) from the park office.

Carbon Canyon Regional Park, on the east fringe of the city of Brea, features only one short hiking trail. Access to the

Chino Hills (east)

Map labels: Bane Canyon Road (main entrance road); Upper Aliso Cyn; Bane Canyon; Raptor Cyn; 850'; Aliso Canyon Trail; RAPTOR RIDGE 1330'; McDermott Trail; Hills for Everyone Trail; Rolling M Ranch (park office); Telegraph Canyon Trail; 1318'; McDermont Spring; South Ridge Trail; 730'; 760'; 1040'; McLean Overlook; Telegraph Canyon Trail; South Ridge Trail; Water Canyon; 1040'; Equestrian Campground; San Juan Hill 1781'; Bobcat Ridge Trail; 675'; CHINO HILLS STATE PARK; Scully Ridge Trail; Brush Canyon; Lower Aliso Canyon; SAN BERNARDINO CO / ORANGE CO; Brush Canyon Trail; 0 0.5 1.0 1.5 miles; 0 0.5 1.0 1.5 km

Chino Hills State Park trail system on this western side is provided by a gateway just east of the regional park entrance and alongside a citrus orchard flanking Carbon Canyon Road.

On the east side, in San Bernardino County, the park has an awkward "main" entrance via gravel and dirt road that was intended to be temporary yet has persisted for many years. To enter that way, exit Highway 71 at Soquel Canyon Parkway (that interchange is 7 miles north of the Riverside Freeway and 5 miles south of the Pomona Freeway). Drive west on Soquel Canyon Parkway 1.0 mile to Elinvar Drive. Turn left, left again after 0.2 mile, and then immediately right on the gravel road signed "Chino Hills State Park." That road, through Bane Canyon,

is open during park hours, 8 A.M. to sunset. After ½ mile you arrive at the park's entrance station. After 2 miles, the road becomes paved and bends sharply right. There's an equestrian campground on the left, and an equestrian staging area with lots of parking space on a knoll to the right. More parking space can be found at the Rolling M Ranch, site of the park office, a little farther ahead along the paved road.

A third designated entrance to Chino Hills State Park can be found at Rim Crest Drive, off Fairmont Boulevard in a suburban neighborhood of Yorba Linda. All other entrances to the state park are indirect and obscure. A separate parcel of land adminstered by Chino Hills State Park lies in lower Coal Canyon, just south

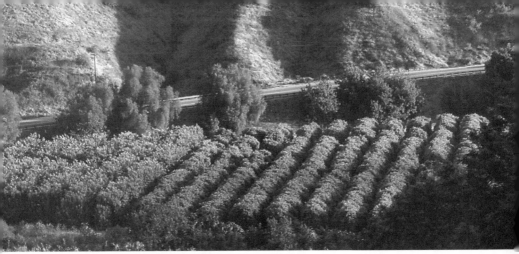

Citrus grove along Carbon Canyon Road

of the Riverside Freeway. The route into that canyon, which lies in the Santa Ana Mountains, is included in Chapter 12, the Santa Ana Mountains—Main Divide section of this book.

For the following trip descriptions, I've selected several shorter hikes in the Chino Hills area, plus a half-day-long, one-way trek across nearly the entire east-to-west dimension of the state park.

TRIP 1 Carbon Canyon Nature Trail

Distance	2.0 miles round trip, Out-and-back
Hiking Time	1 hour (round trip)
Difficulty	Easy
Trail Use	Dogs allowed, good for kids
Best Times	All year
Agency	CCRP
Optional Map	USGS 7.5-min *Yorba Linda*
Notes	Marked trails/obvious routes, easy terrain

DIRECTIONS Exit Highway 57 at Lambert Road in Brea, and drive east. After 2 miles (intersection of Valencia Avenue), Lambert Road becomes Carbon Canyon Road. Continue straight ahead an additional 1 mile to Carbon Canyon Regional Park's entrance on the right (south) side of Carbon Canyon Road.

Carbon Canyon Regional Park, one of the many smaller units of Orange County's far-flung regional park system, has enough room for one significant hiking trail. An unlikely grove of coast redwood trees, nursed from seedlings and planted in 1975, lies at the end of this self-guiding nature trail. Indigenous to the California coast only as far south as Monterey County, their survival in this rather dry corner of Orange County is quite remarkable.

Carbon Canyon Regional Park is a typical suburban recreational facility and features various sports facilities, picnic grounds and pedestrian/bike paths. The entire park lies within the flood zone of the Carbon Canyon flood-control dam, which someday may protect urbanized areas downstream at the expense of inundating the park. The park also happens to lie squarely within the Whittier fault zone, a major splinter of the San Andreas Fault.

The park's nature trail begins just east of the park's entrance. Follow the designated path through a grove of planted pines and down into the bed of Carbon Canyon. The tiny stream is flanked by a variety of water-loving plants: the native mulefat and willow, and the nonnative "giant reed," a naturalized exotic plant resembling bamboo. The reeds tend to compete with native plants for water, and are the target of eradication programs here and elsewhere in Southern California.

After what could be a muddy creek crossing, a trail on the left leads east across a grassy terrace toward Telegraph Canyon in adjoining Chino Hills State Park. Stay right. The nature trail continues west, hugging a dry hillside on the left and dense riparian vegetation on the right. Graceful native walnut trees and nonnative pepper trees can be seen along the hillside, along with nonnative fennel, mustard, and castor bean. The trail bends left into an arm of the basin just above Carbon Canyon dam. Here you find the curious stand of redwoods, a picnic bench, and a drinking fountain. Subsurface water in the basin may keep these redwoods alive, but without the rain and fog drip they are accustomed to in their native habitat, they look a bit thin and dusty.

TRIP 2 Gilman Peak

Distance	7.0 miles round trip, Out-and-back
Hiking Time	3½ hours (round trip)
Elevation Gain/Loss	1400'/1400'
Difficulty	Moderately strenuous
Trail Use	Suitable for mountain biking
Best Times	October through June
Agency	CHSP
Optional Map	USGS 7.5-min *Yorba Linda*
Notes	Marked trails/obvious routes, easy terrain

DIRECTIONS   Exit Highway 57 at Lambert Road in Brea, and drive east. After 2 miles (intersection of Valencia Avenue), Lambert Road becomes Carbon Canyon Road. Continue straight ahead an additional 1 mile to Carbon Canyon Regional Park's entrance on the right. Park your car inside the park for a fee, or outside on the south shoulder of Carbon Canyon for free.

Gilman Peak's bald summit, barely poking over lesser ridges, affords a breathtakingly spacious view of Southern California on a clear day. To the south-west lies the wide mouth of Santa Ana Canyon, scored by a broad flood channel carrying runoff that originates far inland amid the San Bernardino Mountains.

Beyond, the vast urban plain of Orange County, resting on a vast sheet of alluvium, slopes gently toward the ocean. Northward, the gaunt San Gabriel Mountains, snow-capped in winter, rise boldly over foreground hills and valleys. In the southeast, the Santa Ana Mountains form a broad, dusky blister on the horizon.

From the shoulder of Carbon Canyon Road, start hiking or riding on a dirt road slanting southeast, just below the grade of the highway. Following this route, you skirt a citrus orchard (one of the few remaining in Orange County) and soon reach a state park bulletin board at a trail junction. Telegraph Canyon lies ahead; you veer left and start climbing on the North Ridge Trail, a dirt road. There are many California walnut trees to be seen in the next couple of miles, their wispy branches swaying and their compound leaves shimmering in the breeze. These trees, which cling to north-facing slopes, offer welcome shade during the warmer months. They are deciduous, dropping their leaves by the late fall and regaining them in early spring.

By 2 miles into the hike, the trail is staying high on the ridgeline, which is bald save for grass and low-growing sage-scrub vegetation. After you pass over a couple of smaller bumps on the ridge, Gilman Peak appears ahead, its summit accessible by way of a wide side trail from the northeast, and another, narrower side trail from the southwest.

For hikers only (not mountain bikers) it's possible to turn this hike into a loop, by following the no-bikes-allowed Gilman Trail down to Telegraph Canyon and then returning by way of the Telegraph Canyon Trail. Hikers can also reach Gilman Peak by way of trails running north from the Rim Crest Drive trailhead in Yorba Linda. That approach is shorter, but nearly shadeless.

California walnut, a native

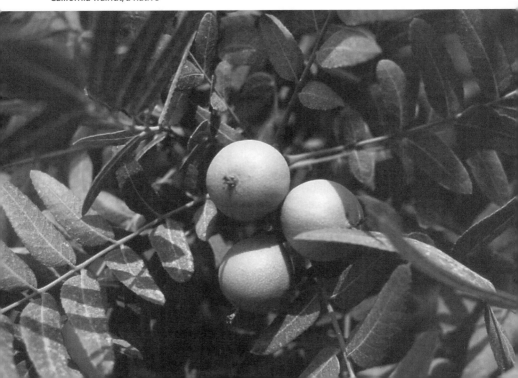

TRIP 3 McLean Overlook

Distance	1.6 miles round trip, Out-and-back
Hiking Time	1 hour (round trip)
Elevation Gain/Loss	300'/300'
Difficulty	Easy
Trail Use	Suitable for mountain biking, good for kids
Best Times	All year
Agency	CHSP
Optional Map	USGS 7.5-min *Prado Dam*
Notes	Marked trails/obvious routes, easy terrain

DIRECTIONS   Exit Highway 71 at Soquel Canyon Parkway in Chino. Drive west on Soquel Canyon Parkway 1.0 mile to Elinvar Drive. Turn left, left again after 0.2 mile, and then immediately right on the gravel road entering Chino Hills State Park. After about 2 miles, where you reach pavement, an old dirt road leading to McLean Overlook appears on the left (east side). Limited parking is here, and plenty more spaces can be found at the large equestrian parking area a short distance ahead.

Worthwhile as an introductory hike, this short stroll takes you to McLean Overlook, a knoll featuring a commanding view of about half of Chino Hills State Park's 13,000 acres.

Start walking up the old road, ignoring a lesser-used road diverging to the left. After 0.4 mile of steep ascent, the road levels out and continues 0.4 mile farther to the overlook. The view encompasses most of the Aliso Canyon drainage. You see rolling, grass-covered hills flanking a shallow valley lined with tall sycamores. In spring the green hills are tinted by the blue-purple flowers of lupine, and accented by yellow bands of blooming wild mustard. Sometime in April or May, quite abruptly, the grass turns a tawny gold. By early fall, after months of fierce sunshine and desiccating winds, it's difficult to believe these same sere hills could ever be green again.

The clayey soils of the hills are derived from bedrock consisting mainly of weak siltstones. These soils expand when wet, and are especially prone to creeping and sliding when waterlogged. You'll notice many examples of recent slumping and gullying on the slopes. Look also for evidence of much older and larger landslides. These big ones probably developed during the last Pleistocene glacial stage (20,000 to 10,000 years ago) when Southern California's climate was much wetter.

Chino Hills

TRIP 4 Upper Aliso Canyon

Distance	3.8 miles, Loop
Hiking Time	2 hours
Elevation Gain/Loss	700'/700'
Difficulty	Moderate
Trail Use	Suitable for mountain biking, good for kids
Best Times	November through May
Agency	CHSP
Optional Map	USGS 7.5-min *Prado Dam*
Notes	Marked trails/obvious routes, easy terrain

DIRECTIONS Exit Highway 71 at Soquel Canyon Parkway in Chino. Drive west on Soquel Canyon Parkway 1.0 mile to Elinvar Drive. Turn left, left again after 0.2 mile, and then immediately right on the gravel road entering Chino Hills State Park. Continue nearly 3 miles to the Rolling M Ranch (park office) at the end of the road, where parking is available.

On this pleasant loop through the upper reaches of Aliso Canyon, you'll appreciate the fine vistas (on clear days at least) of miles of empty hill country presided over by the snow-dusted summits of the San Gabriel Mountains.

From Rolling M Ranch, hike north past outlying staff residences and continue on an old dirt road up the west bank of sycamore-lined Aliso Canyon. At 0.7 mile, the old road passes under some high-voltage wires and soon bends decidedly west up along the bottom of a shallow tributary called Raptor Canyon. A few willows and an occasional walnut tree are all that Raptor Canyon musters for display here.

Upper Aliso Canyon

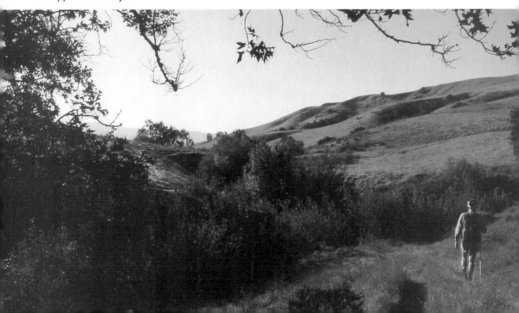

At 1.1 miles, the road veers right and zigzags up the slope to the north. Stay left on the path that strikes west up a grassy ridge just south of Raptor Canyon. After crossing under another power line, you begin a stiff climb of about 500 vertical feet, up through tall-growing grasses, topping out on Raptor Ridge. On the way up, you can look out over the upper reaches of Raptor Canyon, smothered in a rich, dark growth of live oak and walnut trees. True to its namesake, you'll probably notice a hawk or two cruising on updrafts in the canyon.

At 2.0 miles, atop Raptor Ridge, the trail descends a little and you meet a power line access road. Turn left (east), walk 0.3 mile toward a complex of electric towers, and then go right on a road that drops into the wooded drainage to the south. At the bottom (2.8 miles), turn east and return toward your starting point by way of the gently descending Telegraph Canyon Trail (a graded dirt road). When you reach the paved entrance road, turn left and complete the remaining 200 yards back to Rolling M Ranch.

TRIP 5 Hills for Everyone Trail

Distance	5.0 miles round trip (to McDermont Spring), Out-and-back
Hiking Time	2½ hours (round trip)
Elevation Gain/Loss	700'/700'
Difficulty	Moderate
Trail Use	Good for kids
Best Times	October through June
Agency	CHSP
Optional Map	USGS 7.5-min *Prado Dam*
Notes	Marked trails/obvious routes, easy terrain

DIRECTIONS Exit Highway 71 at Soquel Canyon Parkway in Chino. Drive west on Soquel Canyon Parkway 1.0 mile to Elinvar Drive. Turn left, left again after 0.2 mile, and then immediately right on the gravel road entering Chino Hills State Park. Continue nearly 3 miles to the Rolling M Ranch (park office) at the end of the road, where parking is available.

The Hills for Everyone Trail (actually reserved for hikers only—no mountain bikes or equestrian allowed), commemorates "Hills for Everyone," a conservation group that was instrumental in the establishment of Chino Hills State Park. The trail runs up an unnamed tributary of Aliso Canyon, beautifully shaded by live oak, walnut, sycamore, elderberry and toyon.

From the parking lot next to the park office at Rolling M Ranch, walk south on the paved entrance road for about 200 yards, then turn right (west) on the Telegraph Canyon Trail—a maintained dirt road closed to motor traffic. After a near-flat 0.9 mile of travel, look for the Hills for Everyone Trail on the right, going up along the ravine bottom (another, wider trail continues north to Raptor Ridge).

Interpretive panels accompany the trail. For the next 1.3 miles you stick close to the ravine bottom, first on its right, then on its left. During the wet season, water trickles down the bottom, nourishing a moist, dark understory of wild berry vines, ferns, nettles, watercress, and other water-loving plants. Near the top of the trail at 1318 feet, filtered sunlight illuminates wild grape vines draped among the oak trees.

At the top you come to a saddle, part of a major watershed divide. Several trails converge in this area. Raindrops falling to the west are routed down Telegraph Canyon to Carbon Canyon, while rain falling to the east goes into Aliso Canyon. Although most precipitation received in these hills is quickly absorbed by the porous soils, all of the excess eventually makes its way to the Santa Ana River.

Just west of the saddle is McDermont Spring, a small stock pond filled with cattails. Nearby an old windmill groans as it pumps water into a metal tank. Most of the old stock ponds in the park have been allowed to silt up, but this one will be maintained for passing horses and for the benefit of the local wildlife. Look for frogs, pond turtles, and a host of birds in the area hereabouts before you return the same way.

TRIP 6 Water Canyon

Distance	4+ miles round trip, Out-and-back
Hiking Time	2 hours (round trip)
Elevation Gain/Loss	500'/500'
Difficulty	Moderate
Trail Use	Good for kids
Best Times	November through May
Agency	CHSP
Optional Map	USGS 7.5-min *Prado Dam*
Notes	Marked trails/obvious routes, moderate terrain

DIRECTIONS Exit Highway 71 at Soquel Canyon Parkway in Chino. Drive west on Soquel Canyon Parkway 1.0 mile to Elinvar Drive. Turn left, left again after 0.2 mile, and then immediately right on the gravel road entering Chino Hills State Park. Continue about 2 miles to where the entrance road becomes paved. Find space in one of the parking spots along the road, or in the large equestrian staging area near the equestrian campground.

If you're searching for the single most intriguing spot in the Chino Hills, you may find it in the upper reaches of Water Canyon. Concealed in the inky depths of this steep-walled ravine, massive sycamores and oaks reach skyward, casting a perennial chill. Except for the occasional buzz of a small aircraft and the rustle of leaves in the breeze overhead, the silence and stillness are absolute.

From the equestrian campground, start heading south on the wide trail (dirt road) along the shallow valley known as Lower Aliso Canyon. About 0.5 mile from the campground, you dip to cross Aliso Canyon's small stream, which can

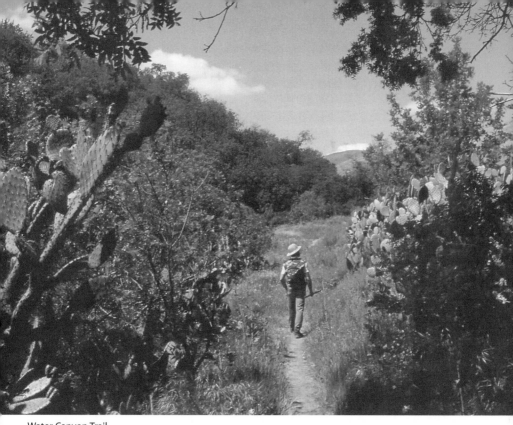

Water Canyon Trail

be wet or dry. On the other side, you join another road at a T-intersection. Turn right, go about 100 yards, and go right again on the narrow trail going up Water Canyon. This is one of the few trails in the park reserved exclusively for hikers. Equestrian and bike traffic is prohibited.

Lining Water Canyon is a narrow finger of riparian willow and sycamore growth, flanked by grizzled oaks and well-proportioned walnut trees. After a short mile you pass a thicket of prickly pear cacti so dense it forms a trailside wall. The trail, which may or not have benefited from recent maintenance, may be partially hidden beyond this point by seasonal grasses, especially after a wet winter season. Intrepid hikers can continue another half mile up along the shady canyon bottom and reach the darkest heart of the canyon, flanked by steep slopes on both sides. Watch out for poison oak, stinging nettles, and rattlesnakes. The pristine little patch of wilderness in upper Water Canyon is as close—and as far—from modern civilization as you will find anywhere around the L.A. metropolitan area.

Chino Hills

TRIP 7 San Juan Hill

Distance	6.4 miles round trip, Out-and-back
Hiking Time	2½ hours (round trip)
Elevation Gain/Loss	1200'/1200'
Difficulty	Moderately strenuous
Trail Use	Suitable for mountain biking
Best Times	November through May
Agency	CHSP
Optional Maps	USGS 7.5-min *Yorba Linda, Prado Dam*
Notes	Marked trails/obvious routes, easy terrain

DIRECTIONS From the intersection of Fairmont and Yorba Linda boulevards in Yorba Linda, drive 1.5 miles north on Fairmont to Rim Crest Drive on the left. Go a short half mile north on Rim Crest to the signed trailhead, on the right. Curbside parking is available here.

A straightforward hike to the high point of Chino Hills State Park, 1781-foot San Juan Hill, can start from either the park office at Rolling M Ranch or the Rim Crest Drive trailhead in Yorba Linda. The latter is a bit longer, but it starts at a point much closer to where most Orange Countians live.

On foot, head uphill a short distance to signed South Ridge Trail (a dirt road). Turn right, heading east along the South Ridge toward San Juan Hill. For 3 miles the trail's gently curling course takes you through a near-treeless landscape. Tall grasses on both sides of the trail sway in the stiff afternoon breezes typically blowing up Santa Ana Canyon from the west. This fact is not lost on kite flyers, who sometimes practice their art here. Keep an eye out for small herds of deer, which roam this section of the park with impunity.

After just over 3 miles of general ascent, take the narrow side trail on the right leading 0.1 mile to the San Juan Hill summit. Nearby high-voltage power lines spoil the view to the east; in other directions, however, the vista is pristine.

TRIP 8 Telegraph Canyon Traverse

Distance	8.2 miles, Point-to-point
Hiking Time	4 hours
Elevation Gain/Loss	650'/900'
Difficulty	Moderately strenuous
Trail Use	Suitable for mountain biking
Best Times	November through May
Agency	CHSP
Optional Maps	USGS 7.5-min *Prado Dam, Yorba Linda*
Notes	Marked trails/obvious routes, easy terrain

DIRECTIONS WEST END: Exit Highway 57 at Lambert Road in Brea, and drive east. After 2 miles (intersection of Valencia Avenue), Lambert Road becomes Carbon Canyon Road. Continue straight ahead an additional 1 mile to Carbon Canyon Regional Park's entrance on the right. Park your car inside the park for a fee, or outside on the south shoulder of Carbon Canyon for free. EAST END: Exit Highway 71 at Soquel Canyon Parkway in Chino. Drive west on Soquel Canyon Parkway 1.0 mile to Elinvar Drive. Turn left, left again after 0.2 mile, and then immediately right on the gravel road entering Chino Hills State Park. Continue nearly 3 miles to the Rolling M Ranch (park office) at the end of the road, where parking is available.

Whether you are hiker, equestrian, or mountain biker, more than 8 miles of superb scenery are yours to enjoy on this one-way trek over the Chino Hills. Telegraph Canyon is long enough, wild enough, and beautiful enough (especially in its upper reaches) to provide a close approximation to a true wilderness experience. Try this trip sometime on a late-autumn afternoon, after the first rains of the season, when the sun's warm rays illuminate the gold and green sycamores, and the cool breeze has a tangy, woodsy aroma.

As in Trip 5, make your way up the Telegraph Canyon Trail and the Hills for Everyone Trail to the saddle, then drop down to McDermont Spring—the headwaters of Telegraph Canyon. (Note: mountain bikes and horses are not allowed on the Hills for Everyone Trail. They must stay on the Telegraph Canyon Trail all the way to the saddle. The dis-tance by that alternate route is only slightly longer.)

Navigational matters are very simple thereafter: just stroll down the bottom of the canyon 5.4 miles until you reach the fringe of the citrus grove at the canyon's mouth. Here, veer right (northwest) toward Carbon Canyon Road and the end of the hike.

Chino Hills

Chapter 7
Foothills:
Santiago Creek/Anaheim Hills

On the eastern fringes of Anaheim and the city of Orange lie several picturesque city and regional (county) parks—all within a half-hour drive of most parts of metropolitan Orange County. This is classic urban-wildland-interface country: suburban housing developments spreading into the foothills of the Santa Ana Mountains, with little beyond but miles of profoundly empty land. In recent years that empty land has been pierced by the Eastern Transportation Corridor toll road—but at the same time most of it has received permanent protection under the umbrella of the Irvine Ranch Land Reserve. That "reserve" consists of 50,000 acres of Irvine Ranch property (over half of the company's historic 93,000-acre cat-

tle ranch) that has or will be deeded to public agencies for use as parkland and open space.

The trips described in this section are found in the following parks: Oak Canyon Nature Center, an Anaheim city park located in that city's Anaheim Hills district; Santiago Oaks Regional Park, east of Villa Park; Weir Canyon Regional Park, an undeveloped buffer of open space just east of Anaheim Hills; Irvine Regional Park, the county's oldest park, located just east of the city of Orange; and the Peters Canyon Regional Park, between Tustin and Orange. In addition to all this, an integrated system of multi-use (hiking, biking, equestrian) trails is slowly taking form in this area and

Black sage on a foggy morning

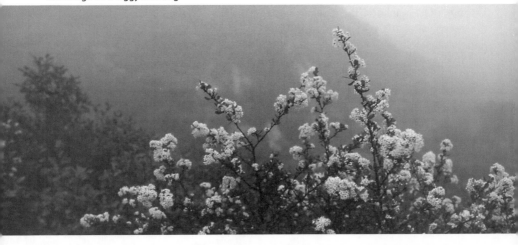

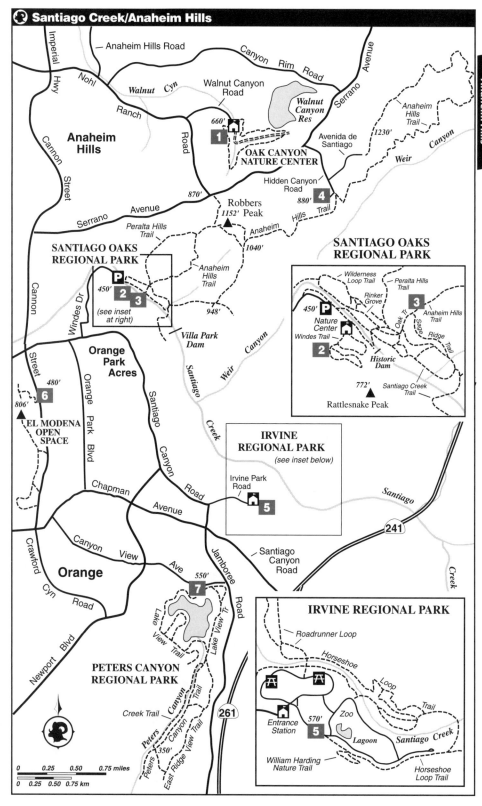

Anaheim Hills Road

Canyon Rim Road

Serrano Avenue

Imperial Hwy

Nohl

Walnut Cyn

Ranch Road

Walnut Canyon Road

660'

1

Walnut Canyon Res

Serrano

Anaheim Hills Trail

1230'

Canyon

Anaheim Hills

Cannon Street

OAK CANYON NATURE CENTER

Avenida de Santiago

Weir

Serrano Avenue

870'

Hidden Canyon Road

880'

4

Anaheim Hills Trail

Robbers 1152' Peak

Peralta Hills Trail

Anaheim Hills Trail

1040'

SANTIAGO OAKS REGIONAL PARK

SANTIAGO OAKS REGIONAL PARK

Cannon

Windes Dr

P

450'

2 **3**

(see inset at right)

Anaheim Hills Trail

948'

Wilderness Loop Trail

Peralta Hills Trail

Rinker Grove

450'

P

3

Nature Center

Oak Tr

Anaheim Hills Trail

Windes Trail

2

Sage Tr

Ridge Trail

Historic Dam

772'

Santiago Creek Trail

Rattlesnake Peak

Villa Park Dam

Weir Canyon

Santiago Creek

Orange Park Acres

Street

480'

6

806'

🔺 **EL MODENA OPEN SPACE**

Orange Park Blvd

Santiago Canyon Road

IRVINE REGIONAL PARK

(see inset below)

Irvine Park Road

5

Santiago

Chapman Avenue

241

Creek

Crawford Cyn Road

Canyon View

Ave

550'

Jamboree Road

Santiago Canyon Road

Orange

7

Lake View Trail

Lake View Tr

IRVINE REGIONAL PARK

Newport Blvd

Roadrunner Loop

Horseshoe

Loop

Trail

🔺

🔺

PETERS CANYON REGIONAL PARK

Peters Canyon Trail

Creek Trail

261

570'

Entrance Station

5

Zoo

Lagoon

Santiago Creek

0   0.25   0.50   0.75 miles
0   0.25   0.50   0.75 km

350'

Peters Canyon Trail

East Ridge View Trail

William Harding Nature Trail

Horseshoe Loop Trail

throughout southern Orange County as well. This "urban" network of city and county trails is designed to link the various regional parks and eventually will tie into the trails of Cleveland National Forest to the east.

TRIP 1 Oak Canyon Nature Center

Distance	1 to 3 miles
Difficulty	Easy
Trail Use	Good for kids
Best Times	All year
Agency	OCNC
Optional Map	USGS 7.5-min *Orange*
Notes	Marked trails/obvious routes, easy terrain

DIRECTIONS Exit the Riverside Freeway (Highway 91) at Imperial Highway in Anaheim Hills. Drive south about ¾ mile to Nohl Ranch Road. Turn left there and go 1.7 miles east to Walnut Canyon Road. Turn left and continue to the end of the road, where abundant free parking is available.

The vest-pocket-sized (58-acre) Oak Canyon Nature Center squeezes between a golf course and a reservoir on one side and a suburban housing tract on the other. Small children have plenty of room to roam on the tightly nested, 4 miles' worth of hiking trails here. It's pretty hard for the little ones to get seriously lost, and the price is right—free. For adults, this is a park to savor slowly. Habitats include a trickling stream shaded by coast live oaks, and hillsides coated with chaparral and sage-scrub vegetation. Following a heavy-rainfall season, the wildflower bloom—especially that of sticky monkeyflower—can be spectacular.

The primary mission of the Oak Canyon Nature Center is education. A slew of workshops and hikes for families and individuals are offered year round. On certain summer evenings there's "Nature Nights"—a twilight walk followed by a presentation in the center's outdoor amphitheater.

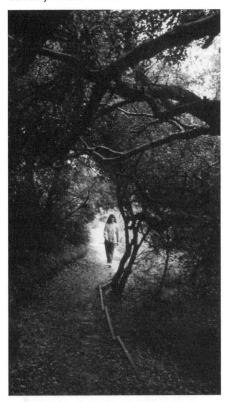
Oak Canyon Nature Center

A few steps from the parking lot will take you to a beautifully rustic interpretive center, nestled under spreading oaks. There you can view some exhibits and pick up a detailed trail map.

On the grounds of the nature center, numerous short trails diverge from the "Main Road," which is a wide path paralleling a small stream in the bottom of Oak Canyon (a tributary of Walnut Canyon). You can go about 0.5 mile to the end of the Main Road, then pick another route for the return. The Stream Trail meanders through the thick of the riparian and oak woodland habitats, while the Roadrunner Ridge and Bluebird trails ascend onto the steep slopes overlooking the ravine bottom. The loop around the outermost perimeter of Oak Canyon Nature Center measures about 2 miles in length.

In summer, you'll find little of interest high on the shadeless, scrub-covered slopes but a lot to enjoy down amid the oaks. In spring, you'll want to gravitate toward the slopes on the south side; this is where a variety of blooming native plants stand shoulder to shoulder.

TRIP 2 Santiago Oaks Regional Park

Distance	1 to 3 miles, Loop
Difficulty	Easy
Trail Use	Dogs allowed, suitable for mountain biking, good for kids
Best Times	All year
Agency	SORP
Optional Map	USGS 7.5-min *Orange*
Notes	Marked trails/obvious routes, easy terrain

DIRECTIONS Exit Highway 55 at Katella Avenue in Orange. Go east on Katella (which quickly become Villa Park Road and finally Santiago Canyon Road) a total of 3 miles to Windes Drive on the left (north). Follow Windes Drive straight into the park.

What Santiago Oaks Regional Park lacks in sheer size is more than adequately compensated for by its rare beauty. The core of the park is made up of two former ranch properties acquired in the mid-1970s. A small Valencia orange grove and many acres of ornamental trees planted around 1960 on these properties complement the natural riparian and oak-woodland communities along Santiago Creek.

As you approach the park entrance on Windes Drive (just north of Santiago Canyon Road), the outlying subdivisions quickly fade from sight and a lush strip of riparian vegetation—willows and sycamores—presided over by steep, scruffy slopes comes into view on the left. Beyond the entrance (day-use fee collected here) and the parking lot, you can stroll up past some oak-shaded picnic sites to the superb nature center which is housed in a nicely refurbished 70-year-old ranch house.

The park is laced with several miles of trail, the best of which stay close to the wooded bottomlands of Santiago Creek. The multi-use trails (hiking, biking, horse riding) stay generally north of Santaigo Creek, while the hiking-only, self-guiding Windes Nature Trail and its Pacifica Loop extension are south of the creek. The 0.7-mile-long Windes Trail plus Pacifica Loop starts at the nature center and meanders very steeply up to the northern summit of Rattlesnake Ridge, an isolated, erosion-resistant block of mostly conglomerate rock. A slice of Pacific coastline can be glimpsed from the high point of the trail, and a fenced lookout point nearby offers a view almost straight down on Santiago Creek and the rest of the park.

Back down by the nature center, you can walk upstream along the shaded creek bank to reach a small rock-and-cement dam dating from 1892. This dam replaced an earlier one, built in 1879, that was part of one of Orange County's first irrigation systems. Today, the surviving dam is a historical curiosity, dwarfed by the large Villa Park flood-control dam a short distance upstream, and Santiago Reservoir farther upstream.

West of the nature center, you can ford Santiago Creek and stroll along several paths amid the eucalyptus, pepper, and other exotic trees rooted to the gently sloping bench on the creek's far side. Because of the diversity of its habitats, Santiago Oaks is a delightful birding spot, with species ranging from the tree-dwelling western bluebird and acorn woodpecker to the water-loving great blue heron. On occasion, vultures and ospreys, as well as some common hawks, may be seen soaring overhead.

Longer-distance trails radiate outward from Santiago Oaks Regional Park toward Irvine Regional Park to the southeast, and up the slopes east and northeast into a county-owned land once dubbed Weir Canyon Regional Park but now incorporated into Santiago Oaks Regional Park. Massive suburban development is taking place on and beyond these slopes—yet thousands of acres in this same area have been designated as permanent open space within the Irvine Ranch Land Reserve.

Santiago Oaks Regional Park

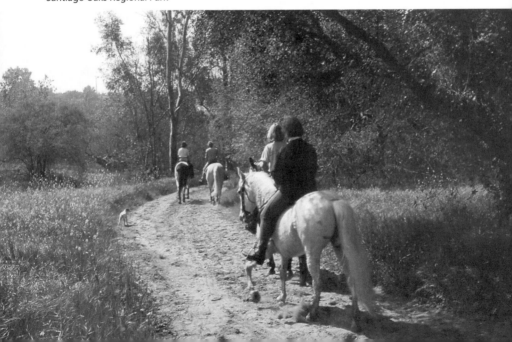

TRIP 3 Robbers Peak

Distance	3.5 miles, Loop
Hiking Time	2 hours
Elevation Gain/Loss	850'/850'
Difficulty	Moderate
Trail Use	Dogs allowed
Best Times	November through May
Agency	SORP
Optional Maps	USGS 7.5-min *Orange*
Notes	Navigation required, moderate terrain

DIRECTIONS Exit Highway 55 at Katella Avenue in Orange. Go east on Katella (which quickly become Villa Park Road and finally Santiago Canyon Road) a total of 3 miles to Windes Drive on the left (north). Follow Windes Drive straight into Santiago Oaks Regional Park, the starting point.

The name Robbers Peak commemorates the notorious outlaws Joaquin Murietta, Three Finger Jack, and others of the late 1800s. Sweeping down out of the hills, these bandits terrorized farmers below and preyed upon passengers traveling the Butterfield Stage. From Robbers Peak they could easily spot and evade sheriff's posses by slipping into the rugged ravines and canyons leading back toward the Santa Ana Mountains.

Whatever historical charm Robbers Peak has is not reflected in the current condition of its summit, which has a sandstone outcrop emblazoned with graffiti. Still, from this height you get a panoramic view of the lowlands to the south and west—a composite of disappearing pastoral landscapes and spreading suburban sprawl. On clear days, the panorama includes the blue arc of the Pacific Ocean and Santa Catalina Island.

There's a trivially easy way to reach Robbers Peak from a public-access gravel roadway starting at Nohl Ranch Road and Serrano Avenue in Anaheim Hills—but the looping route described here is much more scenic and exciting.

Begin hiking at Santiago Oaks Regional Park's parking lot at the end of Windes Road. Cross Santiago Creek at the first opportunity, and continue along the Santiago Creek Trail, with Santiago Creek on your right for 0.6 mile. At that point you reach a trail junction where Santiago Creek Trail continues south, bound for Irvine Regional Park, and the Bobcat Loop trail veers left. Go left, and shortly thereafter find and follow a steep, eroded trail going east up a ridge. As you climb, the massive Villa Park flood-control dam comes into full view, along with its spillway on the far side. At full capacity (that hasn't happened yet), the backup of floodwaters behind this dam would inundate about half of Irvine Regional Park.

At the top of the ridge-running trail (1.1 miles) lies a 948-foot knoll (just west) with the best view yet of the dam and the endless suburbs beyond it. Continue northeast, along the same ridge, which undulates a bit as it climbs toward Robbers Peak. A side trail (the designated Anaheim Hills Trail) intersects at 1.6 miles on the left. Just beyond, in a saddle, the same Anaheim Hills Trail diverges to the right. Keep following the ridge, curling north and then west toward the 1152-foot summit of Robbers Peak, 2.0 miles from the start. North of the summit, new subdivisions press against the sage-dotted hills and canyons. Southward, a big swath of nearly untouched landscape has become a designated part of the Irvine Ranch Land Reserve.

After taking in the view, walk back down the east side of the peak, and turn left on a dirt road heading west just below the peak. You go down along a ridge—taking note of the Anaheim Hills Trail

plunging on the left, and a gravel road branching on the right leading to an elementary school on Serrano Avenue—and proceed to junction with the Peralta Hills Trail (2.5 miles). Stay left on the Anaheim Hills Trail, choosing the more scenic alternative route back down to the starting point. As you descend, Anaheim Hills Trail becomes Oak Trail, and you soon find yourself on the sloping floodplain of Santiago Creek. Use the Rinker Grove Trail paralleling the Santiago Creek Trail, or the Santiago Creek Trail itself, to return to the parking lot.

TRIP 4 Anaheim Hills Trail

Distance	3.7 miles, Loop
Hiking Time	2 hours
Elevation Gain/Loss	500'/500'
Difficulty	Moderate
Trail Use	Good for dogs, suitable for mountain biking, good for kids
Best Times	November through May
Agency	SORP
Optional Maps	USGS 7.5-min *Black Star Canyon*
Notes	Marked trails/obvious routes, easy terrain

DIRECTIONS From the intersection of Serrano Avenue and Hidden Canyon Road (1 mile east of Nohl Ranch Road along Serrano or 2 miles south of Weir Canyon Road along Serrano), turn south on Hidden Canyon Road. After 0.5 mile Overlook Terrace intersects on the right, at the bottom of a hill. Find curbside parking at or near this spot, where there is access to the Anaheim Hills Trail.

The Anaheim Hills Trail (Anaheim Hills Trail System on some maps) skims an undeveloped summit ridge of the Anaheim Hills, drawing significant numbers of hikers, equestrians and mountain bicyclists. The west branch of the trail, the extension of the Oak Trail in Santiago Oaks Regional Park, climbs eastward past Robbers Peak and connects with Hidden Canyon Road in the Ana-

heim Hills section of Anaheim. The east branch, a trail looping northeast, lazily twists and turn along a slope overlooking shallow Weir Canyon and then rises to follow a ridgeline on the second half. This east branch—the most scenic part of the Anaheim Hills Trail—is profiled here.

On foot, proceed on the dirt road going south from Overlook Terrace.

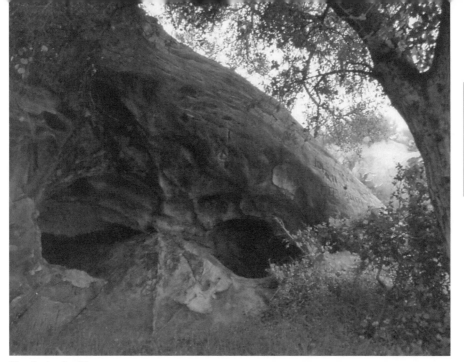

"Eye-Socket Rock"

Immediately there's a split. The right fork is the Anaheim Hills Trail going to Santiago Canyon; the left fork is the looping part of that same trail. Take the left fork and after only 100 yards come to a gate blocking all traffic. Beyond lies Irvine Ranch Land Reserve property that is accessible only on guided tours. Just before this gate, find the narrow trail on the left (Anaheim Hills Trail) and climb up a hill. Immediately to the left you'll spot a pair of closely spaced wind caves carved into a massive outcrop like the vacant eye sockets of a human skull.

For the next 2 miles you follow the crooked course of the trail as it undulates and contours in an out of ravines. The wide floor of Weir Canyon lies below. A rich assemblage of sage-scrub vegetation, dotted here and there with coast live oaks, smothers the slopes hereabouts. Strangely weathered sedimentary strata crop out in many places along the trail, lending an otherworldly feel to the journey—especially when seen in early-morning mist. Throughout these hills and extending higher into the Santa Ana Mountains, outcrops such as these provide nesting sites for swifts, hawks, and other birds. This crooked stretch is fun for kids—though it's good to keep an eye out for mountain bikers, who sometimes tear through here at high speed.

Around 2 miles from the start, the trail climbs, swings sharply left, gains a viewful ridgeline, and follows that ridgeline southwest. Fingers of suburbia reach upward toward the trail on the north.

At 3 miles from the start, the trail pitches downward on the ridgeline. You soon arrive at the east end of a residential street called Avenida de Santiago. Follow that street downhill to where it intersects Hidden Canyon Road, and turn left to reach your starting point.

TRIP 5 Irvine Regional Park

Distance	2 to 4 miles, Loop
Hiking Time	1 to 2 hours
Difficulty	Easy to moderate
Trail Use	Dogs allowed, suitable for mountain biking, good for kids
Best Times	All year
Agency	IRP
Optional Map	USGS 7.5-min *Orange, Black Star Canyon*
Notes	Marked trails/obvious routes, easy terrain

DIRECTIONS From either of the two eastern toll roads (Highways 241 and 261), exit at Santiago Canyon Road. Drive 1 mile northwest to Jamboree Road, and turn right (north). After ¼ mile, stay right on Irvine Park Road, which is the entrance to the park.

For more than a century, Irvine Park has drawn Orange Countians up into the foothills of the Santa Ana Mountains. Once a meeting place for the early settlers—then known as the Picnic Grounds—it became Orange County Park in 1897 when early rancher James Irvine donated 160 acres of prime oak and sycamore groves fronting Santiago Creek. Today's park, now titled Irvine Regional Park, has grown to more than 500 acres and hosts thousands of visitors on busy weekends. The entrance road for the park, on the eastern fringe of the city of Orange, is located at the north end of Jamboree Road.

Aside from picnic and playground areas, a boating lagoon, the small Orange County Zoo, a miniature railroad, and wildlife and historical exhibits—it's possible to find some off-the-beaten-path hiking here. Several miles of paved and unpaved trails suitable for bicycling, hiking, and horse riding follow Santiago Creek and wind around the perimeter of the park. For a nice, short- or medium-length introduction, try this:

Start at the Nature Trail parking area (bear right after passing the entrance station to reach it). Head up the paved path a short distance to the first diversion—the William Harding Nature Area. Here a 0.3-mile self-guiding trail cut into a shady, north-facing hillside introduces you to some of the common chaparral and oak-woodland shrubs and trees.

Continue east along the Horseshoe Loop, which follows the perimeter of the park. At the far east end, bear left and head across Santiago Creek on a concrete crossing. Despite its nearly 100 square miles of drainage, the creek's broad, open bed is almost always dry. This is partly because much of the upstream surface flow has already seeped into porous soils, and partly because Irvine Lake (aka Santiago Reservoir) impounds water upstream. There's still enough water underground, however, to keep the oaks, sycamores and other trees in the park looking healthy. The biggest oaks in the park are as old as 800 years.

On the far side of the creek, keep following the Horseshoe Loop. Before you reach a small outcrop of sandstone, Horseshoe Loop veers right to climb a dry bluff. Continue about 0.4 mile to reach a nearby viewpoint with shade ramada overlooking the green, irrigated

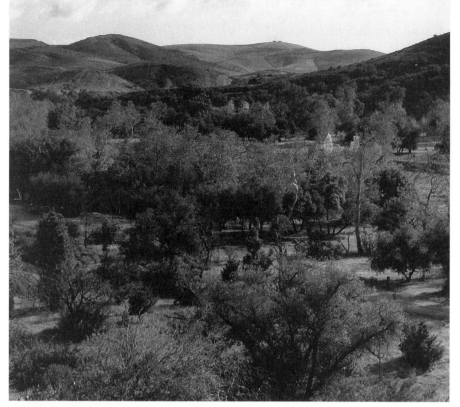

Irvine Regional Park

parts of the park below. This is a good place for a restful pause.

Complete the 2-mile "short-circuit" by descending past the viewpoint into a picnic area below, and then crossing the creekbed via a paved path. Wander among the park's central attractions, clustered around the boating lagoon, to return to the starting point.

For a longer excursion (adding another 2 miles), continue west on Horseshoe Loop 0.5 mile to the Roadrunner Loop. The entire course of the Roadrunner Loop lies on a broad, oak-dotted floodplain alongside Santiago Creek and near the confluence of Weir Canyon. Plenty of groundwater nourishes dense growths of willows and underbrush alongside the creek in this area, providing excellent bird habitat. Bring binoculars!

TRIP 6 El Modena Open Space

Distance	2.4 miles, Loop
Hiking Time	1½ hours
Elevation Gain/Loss	700'/700'
Difficulty	Moderate
Trail Use	Dogs allowed, good for kids
Best Times	All year
Agency	SORP
Optional Maps	USGS 7.5-min *Orange*
Notes	Marked trails/obvious routes, moderate terrain

DIRECTIONS Exit Highway 55 at Chapman Avenue in Orange. Drive 2 miles east to Cannon Street. Turn north and drive 1.3 miles north to Patria Court, on the left, where curbside parking is available.

The long, narrow El Modena Open Space in the city of Orange preserves a steep-sided miniature mountain range, clothed in a tough mixture of drought-resistant cactus and sage-scrub vegetation, and underlain by colorful andesite and pyroclastic rock—volcanic rock dating back some 15 million years. This type of rock, in colors of brick red, pink, white, gray, green and beige, is found in Orange County only here and in a couple of spots just south of Chapman Avenue.

From Cannon Street and Patria Court, follow the path parallel to Cannon's right (southbound) side, and quickly veer right on a steeply ascending trail though a natural garden of California sagebrush, encelia, wild hycinth, and wild onion. As you wind upward toward the top of the ridge, dense thickets of prickly pear cactus, plus some coast cholla cactus, appear.

At the ridgeline turn left and follow it to the highest summit, elevation 806 feet. Enjoy a spacious, pseudo-aerial view of the flat L.A. Basin, wrapping around more than 180 degrees, and the rim of the mountains to the east and north—the Santa Anas and the San Gabriels. This can

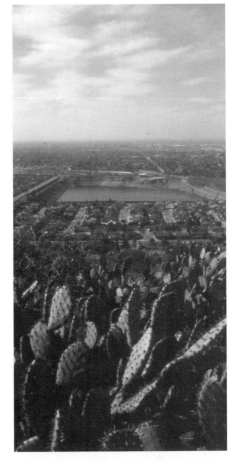
View from El Modena ridgeline

be a mind-blowing view on days of crystalline atmospheric conditions.

From the high point, descend south and pass over two more summits in the next mile. A very steep path goes down the west side of the southernmost hill, and meets a dirt road leading back to the intersection of Cannon Street and Still-water Avenue. Use the bicycle path or sidewalk along Cannon to complete the 1-mile-long return to Patria Court. As done this way, the entire loop measures 2.4 miles.

Two short-cut trails link the ridgeline to Cannon Street, and either one of those can be used to shorten the hike.

TRIP 7 Peters Canyon Regional Park

Distance	3.8 miles (including Creek Trail), Loop
Hiking Time	2 hours
Elevation Gain/Loss	400'/400'
Difficulty	Moderate
Trail Use	Dogs allowed, suitable for mountain biking, good for kids
Best Times	All year
Agency	SORP
Optional Map	USGS 7.5-min *Orange*
Notes	Marked trails/obvious routes, easy terrain

DIRECTIONS From either of the two eastern toll roads (Highways 241 and 261), exit at Santiago Canyon Road. Drive 1 mile northwest to Jamboree Road, and turn left (south). Drive 0.5 mile to Canyon View Avenue, turn right, and then go left into the regional park.

Deeded to Orange County by the Irvine Company in 1992, Peters Canyon Regional Park has, like other newly declared open-space areas, gained almost instant popularity among lovers of the outdoors. The park features the 55-acre Upper Peters Canyon Reservoir, several natural habitats (freshwater marsh, riparian woodland, grassland, and coastal sage-scrub), and about 6 miles of trails. The shallow reservoir is not open to fishing, but birding is fine here. Mats of marsh vegetation and water-loving trees (willows, cottonwoods, and sycamores) hug most of the shoreline, attracting egrets, grebes, herons, and other birds. The park is open from 7 A.M. to sunset daily.

From the park's northern (main) entrance and parking lot, off Canyon View Avenue in the city of Orange, you can start hiking by going west on the Lake View Trail. The shortest circumnavigation of the lake measures less than 2 miles, while side trips to the south, below the reservoir dam, can easily add another 2 miles.

When Lake View Trail meets Peters Canyon Trail, about halfway around the lake, turn right (south) and proceed down the wide Peters Canyon Trail until you reach Creek Trail, which diverges on the right about 300 yards south of the dam. Mountain bikers must stay on the main trail, but hikers can follow the paralleling, relatively primitive Creek Trail.

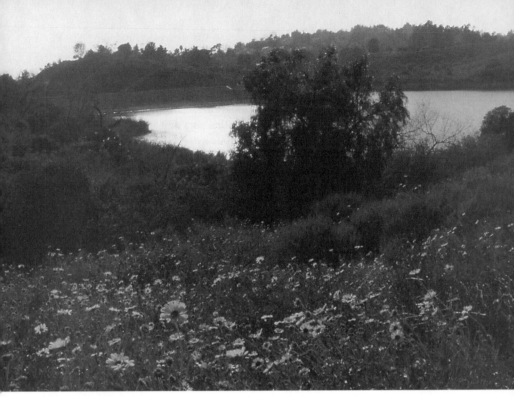

Peters Canyon Reservoir

On it, you duck under the limbs of willow, black cottonwood, and sycamore, inhale the humid odors of riparian vegetation and the pungent scent of eucalyptus, and sometimes (depending on the season) splash through shallow water or squish through mud in the canyon bottom. Footbridges are provided at some of the creek crossings.

At the end of the Creek Trail, you come up out of the shady canyon bottom to join the main Peters Canyon Trail. By turning left, and continuing all the way north on the same trail, you end up circling the reservoir's east side and returning to the starting point.

As you approach the north end of the lake, don't miss the narrow short-cut trail—through a dense growth of willows—on the left. This "Willows Trail" is closed March through September to protect the nesting rights of certain birds.

Chapter 8

Foothills:

Whiting Ranch Wilderness Park

In 1991, Orange County opened the 1500-acre Whiting Ranch Wilderness Park, which sprawls across the foothills of the Santa Ana Mountains just east of the communities of Lake Forest and El Toro. Whiting Ranch's rounded hills look a bit dry and nondescript when viewed from the suburbs below, but up close they reveal some pleasant surprises. One surprise can be found in the upper reaches of a narrow ravine called Borrego Canyon: strangely weathered outcrops of red-tinted sandstone, rising a sheer 100 feet or more. Some people optimistically refer to this natural amphitheater as Orange County's "Little Grand Canyon." The park is also noteworthy for its dense riparian and oak woodland vegetation

which smothers the bottoms of the park's larger ravines.

Whiting Ranch's principal entrance stands alongside a shopping center on Portola Parkway, opposite Market Place and between Alton Parkway and Bake Parkway, east of the Foothill Transportation Corridor toll road in the city of Lake Forest. Look for a trailhead parking lot here, open from 7 A.M. to sunset. Another parking lot serving the park is located on Glenn Ranch Road. A brochure and trail map for the park is available at either trailhead, and maps or directional signs posted at critical trail junctions help make navigation on the trail system easy.

Contiguous parkland in this area will grow dramatically in the next few years as

Trail to The Sinks

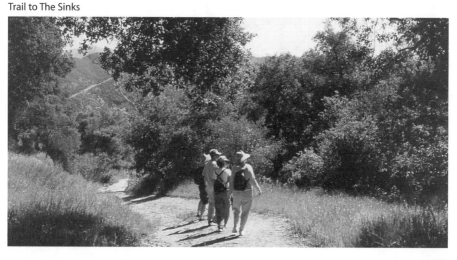

Whiting Ranch
Wilderness Park

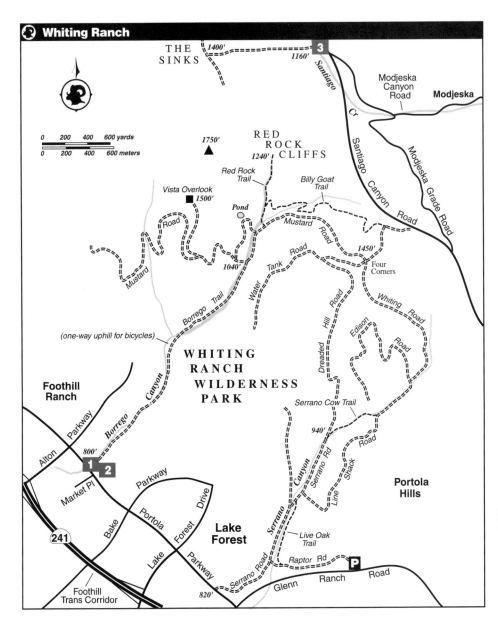

Whiting Ranch

THE
SINKS
1400'
1160'
3

Modjeska
Canyon
Road **Modjeska**

Santiago Cr

0 200 400 600 yards
0 200 400 600 meters

1750'
▲

R E D
R O C K
C L I F F S
1240'

Red Rock
Trail

Billy Goat
Trail

Vista Overlook
■ *1500'*

Pond

Mustard

Road

Santiago Canyon Road

Modjeska Grade Road

Road

1040'

Tank

Water

Borrego Trail

Mustard

1450'

Four
Corners

Whiting Road

(one-way uphill for bicycles)

**WHITING
RANCH
WILDERNESS
PARK**

**Foothill
Ranch**

Canyon

Borrego

Dreaded Hill Road

Edison

Road

Serrano Cow Trail

940'

Road

Parkway

Alton

800'

1 **2**

Market Pl

Parkway

Portola

Bake

Forest Drive

Canyon

Serrano Rd

Line Shack

**Portola
Hills**

(241)

Lake

**Lake
Forest**

Serrano Road

Parkway

Live Oak
Trail

Raptor Rd **P**

Foothill
Trans Corridor

820'

Glenn Ranch Road

Serrano Road

thousands of acres of Irvine Company land to the north pass into public ownership in trade for granting that company certain development rights elsewhere in Orange County. The land immediately north of Whiting Ranch is currently a part of the Irvine Ranch Land Reserve, but is awaiting designation as Limestone Canyon Regional Park. The Nature Conservancy, in cooperation with the Irvine Company and the county parks department, is conducting guided tours of the trails there. One of the most popular of these, a short hike to a dramatic feature called The Sinks, is described in Trip 3.

TRIP 1 Borrego Canyon to Red Rock

Distance	4.0 miles round trip, Out-and-back
Hiking Time	2 hours (round trip)
Elevation Gain/Loss	500'/500'
Difficulty	Moderate
Trail Use	Good for kids
Best Times	October through June
Agency	WRWP
Optional Maps	USGS 7.5-min *El Toro*
Notes	Marked trails/obvious routes, easy terrain

DIRECTIONS Exit the Foothill Transportation Corridor toll road (Highway 241) at Alton Parkway in Lake Forest. Go east on Alton 0.5 mile, turn right on Portola Parkway, and find the trailhead on the left after one long block, opposite Market Place.

From Whiting Ranch's Portola Parkway trailhead, the Borrego Trail leads straightway toward Red Rock canyon, where sandstone cliffs banded with layers of ancient sand and mud rise into the air. The best illumination of the cliffs usually occurs late in the day, when the sun's warm glow brings out the ruddy tint of oxidized iron on the surface of the rock.

Like most trails in the Whiting Ranch Wilderness Park, the Borrego Trail is open to mountain biking and horse riding, as well as hiking. Mountain bikers, however, are not allowed to ride all the way to Red Rock.

At the beginning, you immediately plunge into densely shaded Borrego Canyon, alongside a stream that happily

Borrego Canyon

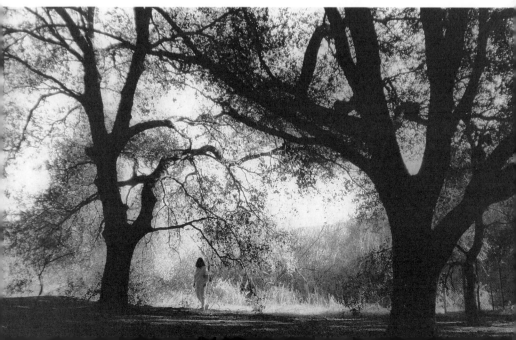

trickles through during winter and spring. For a while, suburbia rims the canyon on both sides, but soon enough it disappears without a trace. The trek up the canyon feels Tolkienesque as you pass under a crooked-limb canopy of live oaks and sycamores, and sniff the damp odor of the streamside willows. Often in the late fall and winter, frigid air sinks into these shady recesses overnight, and by early morning frost mantles everything below eye-level.

After no more than about 40 minutes of walking and 1.3 miles, you come to Mustard Road, a fire road that ascends both east and west to ridgetops offering long views of the ocean on clear days.

Turn right on Mustard Road, pass a picnic site, and take the second trail to the left (the Red Rock Trail—for hikers only), into an upper tributary of Borrego Canyon.

Out in the sunshine now, you meander up the bottom of a sunny ravine that becomes increasingly narrow and steep. Presently, you reach the base of the eroded sandstone cliffs, formed of sediment deposited on a shallow sea bottom about 20 million years ago. This type of rock, which contains the fossilized remains of shellfish and marine mammals, underlies much of Orange County. Rarely is it as well exposed as here.

TRIP 2 Whiting Ranch Loop

Distance	5.5 miles, Loop
Hiking Time	3 hours
Elevation Gain/Loss	800'/800'
Difficulty	Moderately strenuous
Trail Use	Suitable for mountain biking
Best Times	October through May
Agency	WRWP
Optional Map	USGS 7.5-min *El Toro*
Notes	Marked trails/obvious routes, easy terrain

DIRECTIONS Exit the Foothill Transportation Corridor toll road (Highway 241) at Alton Parkway in Lake Forest. Go east on Alton 0.5 mile, turn right on Portola Parkway, and find the trailhead on the left after one long block, opposite Market Place.

For a more comprehensive survey of Whiting Ranch Park, try this circle hike through the park's two largest canyons. You'll travel up Borrego Canyon to a watershed divide, then descend through Serrano Canyon. The basic loop measures 5.5 miles (including a mile on the sidewalk along Portola Parkway at the end), though numerous side trips and extensions are possible if you want to lengthen your hike. If you're mountain biking you must follow the loop in the direction described below, since the initial stretch through Borrego Canyon is designated one-way uphill for bikes.

Start by heading up Borrego Trail from Portola Parkway. At 1.3 miles you meet Mustard Road. Turn right. (To the left, Mustard Road would take you up along grassy slopes to the west, smothered in yellow mustard in the spring). Continue on Mustard Road, going north and later east, up the main tributary of Borrego Canyon to Four Corners (2.2 miles), where four road segments join at a saddle. (A more roundabout way of reaching Four Corners, for hikers only, could involve the Billy Goat Trail, a rough path to the north with constant and often severe ups and downs, and not much shade).

At Four Corners, go across to Whiting Road and start descending—gradually at first along a ridge, then more steeply off the ridge and into an oak-lined valley (upper Serrano Canyon). From now on, simply maintain your descent at all junctions, following the Serrano Cow Trail through a sublime tunnel of live oaks and finally the Serrano Road out to Portola Parkway. From there follow the sidewalk a mile back to your starting point.

TRIP 3 The Sinks

Distance	2.0 miles round trip, Out-and-back
Hiking Time	2 hours or more (on tour)
Elevation Gain/Loss	250'/250'
Difficulty	Easy
Trail Use	Good for kids
Best Times	All year
Agency	TNC
Optional Map	USGS 7.5-min *El Toro*
Notes	Marked trails/obvious routes, easy terrain

DIRECTIONS Participants on the docent-led hike will be instructed to meet along Santiago Canyon Road near Modjeska Canyon. Reservations are required.

The 5500-acre Limestone Canyon parcel of the Irvine Ranch Land Reserve awaits its future as a fully accessible wilderness park, much like the adjacent Whiting Ranch Wilderness Park is today. Meanwhile, The Nature Conservancy sponsors hiking, equestrian, and mountain biking tours of the property, ranging in length from 2 miles to 15 miles. The most popular tour of all, the easy hike to The Sinks, is a "must-have" experience for O.C. hikers. Those who have already had the experience in the daytime can repeat it during scheduled full-moon evening tours, which are given nearly every month.

Contact The Nature Conservancy at (714) 832-7478 or e-mail irvineranch@ tnc.org for a tour schedule and reservation instructions. Participants may gather at a staging area elsewhere and then be shuttled to or carpool to the limited-parking trailhead, which lies along Santiago Canyon Road, north of Modjeska.

Starting your hike from there, you begin by crossing the wide, bouldery bed of Santiago Creek and picking up a dirt road heading up a small canyon on the far side. Graced with shade-giving live oaks and lush riparian vegetation, the canyon is recovering from a century or more of cattle-grazing use. Expect progress to be slow; your guide will likely point out every significant type of plant, and spin yarns about various birds and animals that may come into view.

At 0.8 mile you reach the head of the small canyon, where you meet a ridge-running dirt road. You turn north and continue about 0.2 mile to the best viewpoints overlooking the steep-walled sandstone gorge named The Sinks. Erosion of the soft sedimentary rock here has led to the formation of a receding cliff—most dramatically sheer on the north side, where it exhibits a relief of about 150 feet. The scene is impressive under mid-morning sunlight, and spectacular in bright moonlight.

The Sinks

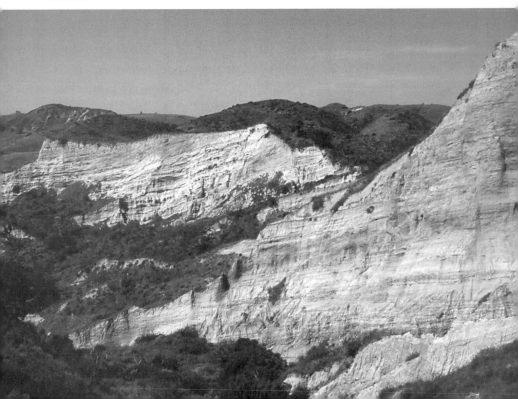

Chapter 9
Foothills:
O'Neill Regional Park/Mission Viejo

Encompassing more than 3000 acres of riparian bottomlands, oak woodlands, grassy meadows, and scrub-covered hills, O'Neill Regional Park is one of the oldest parks in Orange County. Starting with 278 acres donated in 1948 by the descendants of the O'Neill family (owners of what was once a vast ranching empire stretching across southern Orange County), the park grew steadily to accommodate the needs of the expanding county population. A nice complement of recreational facilities was developed: picnic tables, a playground, a ball field, a small arboretum, and camping areas for equestrians and motorists. Later additions to the park west of Live Oak Canyon Road made possible the development of an extensive trail system for hikers, horseback riders, and mountain bikers.

The most recent acquisition, the 935-acre Arroyo Trabuco Wilderness, laid off-limits for more than a decade before it opened for public use in 1995. Its long, curvilinear form, stretching almost 6 miles through the suburban landscape of Mission Viejo, serves as an important wildlife corridor between the Santa Ana Mountains and the remaining open spaces of coastal Orange County. This and other long, narrow strips of open space throughout this growing part of the county are being preserved in perpetuity as greenbelts.

South of O'Neill Park, another patch of open space, laden with trails, welcomes you. This 475-acre parcel, Thomas F. Riley Wilderness Park, was deeded to the county in 1983 by the developers of the adjacent community of Coto de Caza. Not until easy access was assured (by way of the east extension of Oso Parkway) was the park opened for public use in December 1994. The Riley Park trails are described in Trip 3 of this section.

A fourth trip in this section, new to the current edition of this book, is the Bell View Regional Trail, one of several long-distance trails in the county designed to tie together various parks and open space areas. The Bell View Trail threads the boundary between suburbs to the west and wildland to the east, beginning in Rancho Santa Margarita and ending at Caspers Wilderness Park.

O'Neill Regional Park/
Mission Viejo

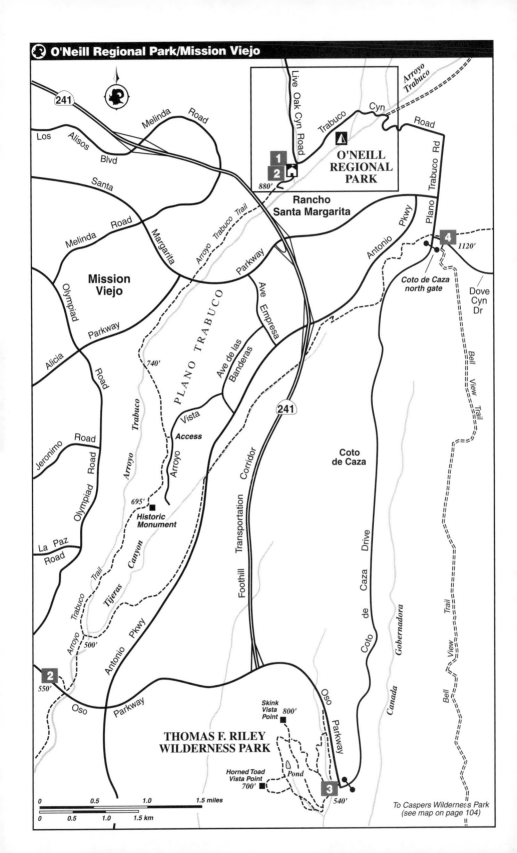

241

Live Oak Cyn Road

Arroyo Trabuco

Melinda Road

Trabuco Cyn Road

Los Alisos Blvd

1
2

880'

O'NEILL REGIONAL PARK

Plano Trabuco Rd

Santa Road

Rancho Santa Margarita

Arroyo Trabuco Trail

Antonio Pkwy

4
1120'

Melinda Road

Margarita

Parkway

Mission Viejo

Ave Empresa

Coto de Caza north gate

Dove Cyn Dr

Olympiad Parkway

Bell View Trail

Alicia

P L A N O   T R A B U C O

740'

Ave de las Banderas

241

Jeronimo Road

Olympiad Road

Arroyo Trabuco

Arroyo

Vista

Access

Transportation Corridor

Coto de Caza

695'
■
Historic Monument

Canyon

Foothill

Coto de Caza Drive

Gobernadora

Bell View Trail

La Paz Road

Tijeras Trail

Antonio Pkwy

500'

Canada

2
550'

Oso Parkway

THOMAS F. RILEY WILDERNESS PARK

Skink Vista Point
800' ■

Oso Parkway

Horned Toad Vista Point
700' ■

Pond

3
540'

0   0.5   1.0   1.5 miles
0   0.5   1.0   1.5 km

To Caspers Wilderness Park (see map on page 104)

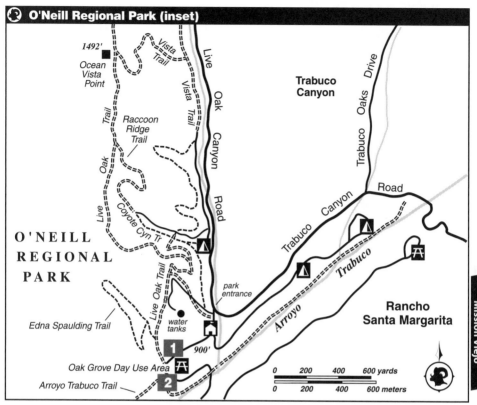

O'Neill Regional Park (inset)

1492'
Ocean Vista Point

Vista Trail

Live Oak Canyon Road

Trabuco Canyon

Trabuco Oaks Drive

Raccoon Ridge Trail

Oak Trail

Live Oak Trail

Coyote Cyn Tr

O'NEILL REGIONAL PARK

Edna Spaulding Trail

water tanks

900'

Oak Grove Day Use Area

Arroyo Trabuco Trail

park entrance

Trabuco Canyon Road

Arroyo Trabuco

Rancho Santa Margarita

0   200   400   600 yards
0   200   400   600 meters

TRIP 1 Ocean Vista Point

Distance	3.2 miles, Loop
Hiking Time	1½ hours
Elevation Gain/Loss	650'/650'
Difficulty	Moderate
Trail Use	Dogs allowed, suitable for mountain biking, good for kids
Best Times	All year
Agency	ONRP
Optional Map	USGS 7.5-min *Santiago Peak*
Notes	Marked trails/obvious routes, easy terrain

DIRECTIONS Drive south on Live Oak Canyon Road from where it joins with El Toro Road and Santiago Canyon Road (Cook's Corner). Continue for 3 miles to the O'Neill Regional Park entrance, and park inside at the Oak Grove day-use area.

An inspiring vista of sea on one side, and chaparral- and sage-covered mountains on the other, awaits you at the mid-point of this hike, a 1492-foot-high overlook in O'Neill Regional Park. Don't forget binoculars and perhaps a county

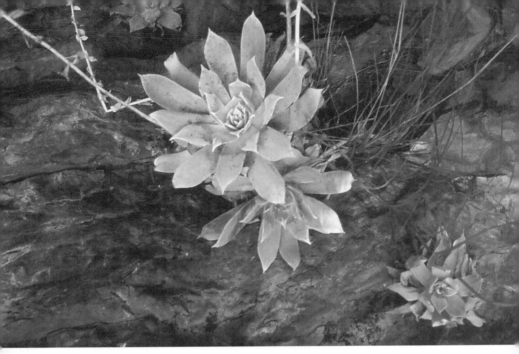

Live-forever plants

map to familiarize yourself with Orange County's urban and natural geography.

From the Oak Grove day-use area, pick up the Live Oak Trail, which heads north and upward onto a dry slope. Ignoring the Edna Spaulding Trail on the left, pass under a couple of hilltop water tanks, and for a moment touch upon the paved driveway going to those tanks. Stay left on the ascending Live Oak Trail, swing around two hairpin turns, and stay left at the next fork, remaining on Live Oak Trail. You climb up to and then along the top of a viewful ridgeline. Your destination, a 1492-foot bump on the ridge ahead called the "Overlook" on park maps, may be identified from afar by a spiky cellular-telephone antenna structure near its top.

Breezy days from late fall to early spring are best for the Overlook's view. Often visible above the layer of low haze or smog are San Clemente and Santa Catalina islands, the Palos Verdes Peninsula, and the Santa Monica Mountains. To the east, the Santa Ana Mountains rise impressively—so much more so because you look down on their lower flanks, as well as up to their summits.

To make this hike a loop trip and to return quickly, drop east on the Vista Trail toward shady Live Oak Canyon. Bear right at the bottom and follow an old, mostly paved service road paralleling Live Oak Canyon Road. Continue south (very gradually downhill) until you reach your starting point.

TRIP 2 Arroyo Trabuco

Distance	5.8 miles, Point-to-point
Hiking Time	3 hours
Elevation Gain/Loss	170'/500'
Difficulty	Moderately strenuous
Trail Use	Dogs allowed, suitable for mountain biking
Best Times	October through June
Agency	ONRP
Optional Maps	USGS 7.5-min *Santiago Peak, Canada Gobernadora, San Juan Capistrano*
Notes	Marked trails/obvious routes, easy terrain

DIRECTIONS NORTH END (starting point): Drive south on Live Oak Canyon Road from where it joins with El Toro Road and Santiago Canyon Road (Cook's Corner). Continue for 3 miles to the O'Neill Regional Park entrance. SOUTH END (pick-up point): Oso Parkway, 2 miles east of Interstate 5 and 0.3 mile west of Antonio Parkway (on the west end of Oso Parkway's long bridge over Arroyo Trabuco.

The somewhat long but easy-going trek down the Arroyo Trabuco is most adventurous after winter rainy periods, when turbid water dances over a wide, gravelly bed, and there's no way to avoid a good foot-soaking at each of four fords you encounter along the trail. Be aware, however, that for most county-park trails such as this, there's usually a "drying-out" period (usually 3 days) during which all visitation is prohibited.

By early April, waist-high green grass pokes upward from the soft ground and the emerging leaves on the sycamores flutter on the marine air that persistently pushes its way inland. Blooming mustard and poppies appear as April grades into May—just as the grass bleaches to yellow or brown. By summer the arroyo creekbed is usually dry, and the midday heat can be oppressive. The scenery improves greatly in November and December as the sycamore leaves turn crispy and yellow and drift earthward on capricious puffs of Santa Ana wind.

Begin at the west end of the Oak Grove day-use area, west of the O'Neill Park office, where the well-marked trail down along the Arroyo Trabuco begins. You soon pass under a massive twin bridge (Foothill Transportation Corridor toll road) and later pass under another equally huge bridge (Santa Margarita Parkway). As an environmental mitigation for the construction of these bridges, county workers and volunteers have planted on the arroyo banks thousands of native trees and shrubs—live oak, sycamore, toyon, mulefat, and willow. Barring huge floods, this upper stretch of the arroyo will look more lush with the passage of time.

At 1.9 miles, well past the second bridge, the trail swings left across the creek and ascends moderately toward the lip of the shallow gorge and toward a subdivision built upon the sloping plain to the east, called Plano Trabuco. The plano ("plain" in English) is a broad terrace made up of alluvial deposits cast off of the Santa Ana Mountains. Over recent geologic time, the abrasive floodwaters of Arroyo Trabuco have cut about 100 feet deep into Plano Trabuco's soft sediments.

O'Neill Regional Park / Mission Viejo

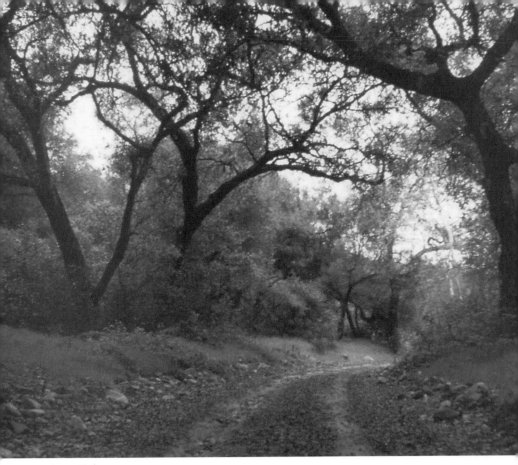

Arroyo Trabuco

Plano Trabuco acquired its name in 1769, when a soldier traveling with the Portola expedition lost a blunderbuss (trabuco) there. A string of contemporary place names are descended from the original: Arroyo Trabuco, Trabuco Canyon, and the Trabuco Ranger District—the part of Cleveland National Forest that encompasses the Santa Ana Mountains.

After a moderate ascent, the Arroyo Trabuco Trail sidles up to a residential street called Arroyo Vista, where there is a signed access point for the trail. Plenty of curbside parking is here, if you want to plan a shorter trip up or down the arroyo. A mile farther, the trail descends back into the gorge. On the left, before you begin the descent, notice a small structure accompanied by a historical plaque. This marks the campsite, designated San Fran-cisco Solano, used by the Portola expedition on the night of July 24–25, 1769.

After the descent, the trail continues for another 2 miles down alongside the wide floodplain, always staying close to the streambed. This is perhaps the most agreeable part of the arroyo, with gnarled sycamores and oaks alternating with grassy clearings. After three stream crossings, the Oso Parkway bridge looms high overhead. Underneath it you can pick up a powerline access road up the right (west) slope of the arroyo, and ascend to reach the shoulder of Oso Parkway.

TRIP 3 Riley Wilderness Park

Distance	3.0 miles, Loop
Hiking Time	1½ hours
Elevation Gain/Loss	350'/350'
Difficulty	Moderate
Trail Use	Good for kids
Best Times	All year
Agency	RWP
Optional Maps	USGS 7.5-min *Canada Gobernadora*
Notes	Marked trails/obvious routes, easy terrain

DIRECTIONS Find the Riley Park entrance at the end of Oso Parkway, 2 miles east of the Foothill Transportation Corridor toll road and 6 miles east of Interstate 5.

Thomas F. Riley Wilderness Park, a wilderness in name only, spreads over 475 acres of rolling hills and oak-lined ravines, and includes about 5 miles of trails open to hikers, equestrians, and mountain bikers. Like much of Orange County's foothills, this area was until recently home to far more cattle than people. Hardly pristine in a biological sense, the park nonetheless preserves a nice pocket of open space that will permanently resist the bulldozer blade. A vast stretch of land to the north and east is being transformed into suburban and rural housing, and by perhaps 2008 the Foothill Transportation Corridor toll road will be extended south along the west edge of the park.

The following moderately easy trek around the park's perimeter is rewarding for hikers (mountain bikers must stick to a more limited subset of multi-use trails.) From the parking lot, head north on oak-shaded Wagon Wheel Canyon Trail, which runs parallel to Oso Parkway. After 0.4 mile, turn left, cross the shallow bottom of Wagon Wheel Canyon, and double back south on the narrow Pheasant

Wagon Wheel Canyon

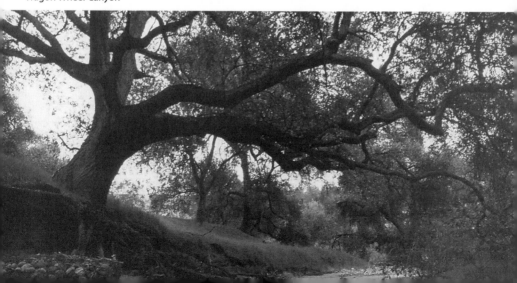

O'Neill Regional Park / Mission Viejo

Run Trail. After a gentle rise and a fall you arrive at the Mule Deer Trail, nearly back at the starting point. Make a sharp right and start climbing again. Early spring brings forth a good display of wildflowers on the grassy hillsides ahead: shooting stars, lupine, wild hyacinth, and monkeyflower. Later in the spring, blooming mustard paints yellow patches across these slopes.

The crooked climb on the Mule Deer Trail leads toward a ridgetop trail junction. Skink Vista Point, offering a somewhat wider view of the park and its surroundings, lies on the bald ridgeline a little higher and farther north of that junction. Jog left a little and turn right, starting a short and sharp descent into a shallow valley. Proceed south down the valley past a old stock pond, noting the sign for Horned Toad Vista Point on the right. The short and steep side trip up through aromatic sage-scrub vegetation is worth it; from the top of the trail you can gaze down on the most secluded parts of the park.

Returning to the previous trail, turn right and descend toward the oak- and sycamore-dotted floor of the valley. By staying right at all subsequent junctions you will return to the parking lot, approaching it from the south.

TRIP 4 Bell View Trail

Distance	8.5 miles (to windmill at Caspers), Point-to-point
Hiking Time	4 hours
Elevation Gain/Loss	1000'/1650'
Difficulty	Moderately strenuous
Trail Use	Suitable for mountain biking
Best Times	November through May
Agency	CWP
Optional Maps	USGS 7.5-min *Santiago Peak, Canada Gobernadora*
Notes	Marked trails/obvious routes, easy terrain

DIRECTIONS NORTH END: Exit the Foothill Transportation Corridor toll road (Highway 241) at Santa Margarita Parkway. Proceed east 1.7 miles to Plano Trabuco Road. Turn right, go 0.4 mile, and find parking space at or near Plano Trabuco Road and Dove Canyon Drive. SOUTH END: Exit Interstate 5 at Ortega Highway (Highway 74) in San Juan Capistrano. Proceed east 7.6 miles to Caspers Wilderness Park on the left.

The Bell View Regional Trail, for hikers, equestrians, and cyclists, starts as a "community trail" threading through the suburban-edge communities of Rancho Santa Margarita and Coto de Caza. It then assumes a wilder character as it undulates along a ridge overlooking open land to the east as far as the eye can see. The route ends inside Caspers Wilderness Park, not far from Ortega Highway. For mountain bikers, the out-and-back distance of 17+ miles seems reasonable. Hikers, however, will better enjoy the journey as an 8.5-mile point-to-point hike facilitated by a willing driver-friend. Arrange to have your friend drop you off at the start, the north gate for the private Coto de Caza housing development, and pick you up at the finish, either the historic windmill site or the Old Corral Picnic Area. By car, the shortest distance between start and end points of this route is about 15 miles by way of Antonio Parkway and Ortega Highway. That driving distance will be shortened when the Foothill Transportation Corridor toll road is extended to as far as Ortega Highway.

The Bell View Trail begins on a paved service road just east of a faux waterfall, which is part of the Dove Canyon housing development entrance. Head south up a short, steep hill on the service road, and then veer right on the decomposed-granite path designated the Bell View Trail. You climb toward a broad ridge, with Coto de Caza houses stretching miles ahead down the valley on your right, and the Dove Canyon subdivision and golf course to your left (east).

After 2 miles of unexciting travel, you descend past the last of the Dove Canyon

housing and pick up an old dirt road alongside the east boundary of the spacious (and closed to the public except for special tours) Audubon Society Starr Ranch Sanctuary. A sign indicates that dogs are not allowed on the trail anywhere south of this point.

At 2.6 miles you pass an equestrian rest area with a drinking fountain and picnic tables. Continue south, on or near the top of the ridgeline, occasionally going steeply up or down. The Coto de Caza development continues on the right side, while the Bell Canyon drainage lies on the left. Note the effect of regional uplift in this area over a period of a million years or so. The shelf-like fluvial (stream) terraces flanking the canyon represent where the river once flowed across a broad plain. The brooding Santa Ana Mountain rise in back of this spacious scene, with no sign of civilization in that direction.

Resting bench overlooking Bell Canyon

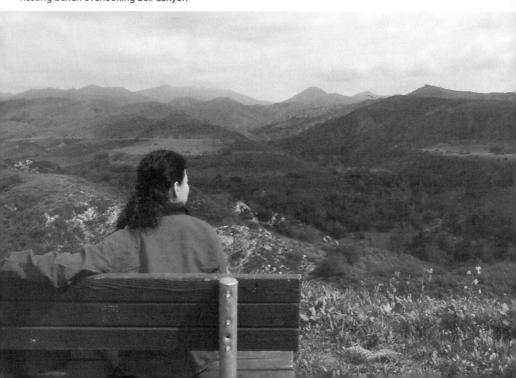

At 3.8 miles you reach a gate. Go around it and bear left to stay on the Bell View Trail. The trail follows for a time one of the flat terraces, which at this point lies on the ridgeline, then descends to the west side, passing assorted ruins of the not-long-bygone cattle-ranching era. At 5.2 miles there's bench with a view down into Bell Canyon. The name "Bell," incidentally, commemorates an eight-ton granitic boulder, scored with mazelike petroglyphs, that once lay precariously balanced on some smaller rocks in what is now the Audubon Sanctuary. When struck with great force, the boulder resonated like a bell, audible a mile away. Removed from the canyon in 1936, Bell Rock was taken to the courtyard of the Bowers Museum in Santa Ana, where it rests today.

Just ahead of the resting bench, a sign announces your arrival at Caspers Wilderness Park. Continue 2.2 miles down the ridge-running road (now called the West Ridge Trail) to a junction with Star Rise, a fire road descending east into Bell Canyon. Make a left, descend to the bottom, and make a right on Oak Trail. Continue for short mile on the delightfully woodsy Oak Trail, which meanders through oak and sycamore woodland on the left or west bank of Bell Canyon. Just before arriving at the end, you'll encounter the Nature Trail Loop. Go left to reach the Old Corral Picnic Area or stay right to reach the historic windmill site. (Note: mountain bikers must stay on Star Rise as it swings north and connects with Bell Canyon Trail. The Oak and Nature Loop trails are off-limits to bikes.)

Chapter 10
Foothills:
Caspers Wilderness Park

Caspers Wilderness Park is without a doubt the crown jewel of Orange County's regional (county) park system. It is the largest park established to date in the county, the least altered by human activities, and the most remote from population centers. Its position adjacent to Cleveland National Forest on the east and north, and the Audubon Society's Starr Ranch Sanctuary on the north and west, integrates it into the only good-sized area within Orange County that could truthfully be called a wilderness. Caspers wouldn't qualify as a statutory wilderness (that is, roadless and primitive) area by federal standards, as does nearby San Mateo Canyon Wilderness, but the richness of its wildlife is testimony enough to its de facto primitive state.

Strangely enough, the area encompassing Caspers Park—the former Starr Ranch—narrowly escaped development as a commercial amusement park back in the early 1970s. Fortunately, the owners of the property at the time went bankrupt. Instead, most of the north half of the property was deeded to the Audubon Society in 1973. The south half was purchased by Orange County in 1974 for use as a regional park, largely through the efforts of Board of Supervisors chairman Ronald W. Caspers. Subsequent purchases increased the total park area to its present 8000 acres.

True to the vision of those who foresaw Caspers Park as protecting one of Orange County's last natural areas and as being a great recreation resource as well,

Juaneno Trail, Caspers Park

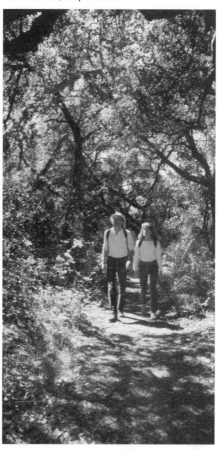

103

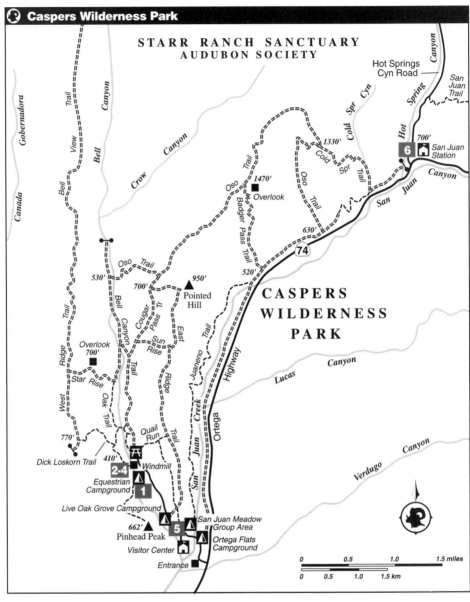

the park today is graced with a fine complement of facilities and improvements. The beautiful visitor center houses a small museum and an open-air loft offering spectacular views of the Santa Ana Mountains. The camping and picnic facilities are second to none in Orange County; a separate area is included for equestrians. Radiating out to the outer reaches of the park are 35 miles of riding and hiking trails.

Protection and enhancement of natural habitat are among the park's most important goals. To this end firebreaks have been constructed on some of the ridges in order to facilitate controlled burns. Periodic burning favors native plants over the non-native grasses and weedy plants introduced in the past, and helps to maintain the natural sage-scrub vegetation, which is well adapted to fire. Parts of these firebreaks have been incorporated into the trail system, which also includes dirt maintenance roads and footpaths. A firestorm in October 1993 (one of several simultaneous fires that burned throughout Southern California) swept the northeastern two-thirds of the park, but did not destroy any of the park's visitor facilities.

Several days could be spent exploring the remainder of the trail system, which visits two basic kinds of environments: (1) the always impressive oak-and-sycamore woodlands along San Juan and Bell canyons (the two largest drainages in the park); and (2) the sage- and chaparral-covered hillsides offering at times magnificent views stretching from the ocean to the Santa Ana Mountains. You can start with one of the following.

TRIP 1 Pinhead Peak

Distance	1.5 miles round trip, Out-and-back
Hiking Time	1 hour (round trip)
Elevation Gain/Loss	400'/400'
Difficulty	Easy
Trail Use	Good for kids
Best Times	All year
Agency	CWP
Optional Map	USGS 7.5-min *Canada Gobernadora*
Notes	Marked trails/obvious routes, easy terrain

DIRECTIONS Exit Interstate 5 at Ortega Highway (Highway 74) in San Juan Capistrano. Proceed east 7.6 miles to Caspers Wilderness Park on the left.

The view from the visitor center is impressive, but from Pinhead Peak it's even better. Here you can look down on the three-way confluence of dry creekbeds—San Juan, Bell, and Verdugo—and spot the toylike visitor center perched atop the knoll between the first two.

You may pick up the trail, for hikers only, at either the Starr Mesa Equestrian Campground, or the historic windmill a little farther north. Travel south across a meadow into a grassy cove, then follow a better-defined trail up onto the scrub-covered ridge on the left. After a short but vigorous climb, you'll reach a high point

on the ridge next to a wire fence defining the park boundary. This is the 662-foot peak called "Pinhead." The trail continues 200 yards to a slightly lower bump on the ridge offering a more panoramic view. From both peaks almost the entire extent of Caspers Park can be seen. Successively higher ridges lead the eye northward and eastward toward the two summits of Old Saddleback and other notable promontories in the southern Santa Ana Mountains.

Caspers Wilderness Park

TRIP 2 Oak Trail Loop

Distance	2.8 miles, Loop
Hiking Time	1½ hours
Elevation Gain/Loss	200'/200'
Difficulty	Easy
Trail Use	Good for kids
Best Times	All year
Agency	CWP
Optional Map	USGS 7.5-min *Canada Gobernadora*
Notes	Marked trails/obvious routes, easy terrain

DIRECTIONS Exit Interstate 5 at Ortega Highway (Highway 74) in San Juan Capistrano. Proceed east 7.6 miles to Caspers Wilderness Park on the left.

Magnificent coast live oak trees, the largest in the park, line this trail along the west side of Bell Canyon. The Spanish called this tree *la encina*, a word whose derivatives are echoed in the communities of Encino near Los Angeles and Encinitas ("little oaks") near San Diego.

Start at the historic windmill (a mile north by paved road from the visitor center), following the hiking/equestrian Nature Trail Loop. Cross the gravelly bed of Bell Canyon and stay on the far side for the next 1.0 mile, using the Nature Trail loop at first, then the north-trending Oak Trail.

As if stricken with some kind of arboreal arthritis, the limbs and branches of the oaks are fantastically contorted. Actually there's an underlying order to the seemingly random pattern. By intricately branching, the tree can support more leaves with less wood. Many of the oaks show fire scars dating back to the Stewart fire of 1958, which originated in Riverside County. Pushed along by Santa Ana winds, the fire swept across all of what is now Caspers Park, charring a total of 66,000 acres. This area was not quite reached by the 1993 fire, which also swept

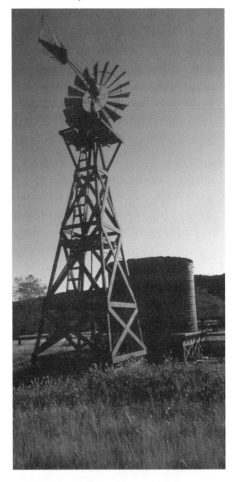

Windmill at Caspers Park

southwest on a Santa Ana, but stalled about a mile from here.

In late fall the tall sycamores along the Oak Trail can be even more attractive than the oaks. Crunch through the crispy leaf litter beneath their spreading crowns and watch the golden sunbeams dance amid thousands of fluttering leaves overhead. In winter the trunks and branches are ghostly white. By early spring, new leaves are emerging, and sunlight passing though them bathes the ground shadows in a jungle-green luminance.

When you reach Star Rise (the fire road coming down from Bell Canyon's west ridge) turn right. After proceeding north along Star Rise for 0.4 mile, you reach Bell Canyon Trail. Turn right, continue up and over a little hill, and remain on the gradually descending Bell Canyon Trail for the remainder of the hike.

TRIP 3 West Ridge-Bell Canyon Loop

Distance	3.3 miles, Loop
Hiking Time	1½ hours
Elevation Gain/Loss	400'/400'
Difficulty	Moderate
Trail Use	Good for kids
Best Times	October through June
Agency	CWP
Optional Map	USGS 7.5-min *Canada Gobernadora*
Notes	Marked trails/obvious routes, easy terrain

DIRECTIONS Exit Interstate 5 at Ortega Highway (Highway 74) in San Juan Capistrano. Proceed east 7.6 miles to Caspers Wilderness Park on the left.

This hike features a rather dizzying passage across the top of some curious white sandstone formations, rather like the breaks along the upper Missouri River or the barren cliffs of the South Dakota badlands. You'll loop up and over the main ridge defining the west edge of the park, enjoying views of adjacent areas of the county not ordinarily seen from any road.

Begin hiking at the historic windmill (a mile north by paved road from the visitor center) on the Nature Trail Loop. Follow that path across the wide bed of Bell Canyon and into the dense oak woodland on the far side. After 0.3 mile you'll spot a park bench beneath a gorgeous, spreading oak tree. A little farther on, veer left on the Dick Loskorn Trail. This path meanders up a shallow draw and soon climbs to a sandstone ridgeline that at one point narrows to near-knife-edge width. At one point you step within a foot of a modest but unnerving abyss. The sandstone is part of a marine sedimentary formation, called the Santiago Formation (roughly 45 million years old), which crops out along the coastal strip from here down to mid-San Diego County.

After climbing about 350 feet, you come to a dirt road—the West Ridge

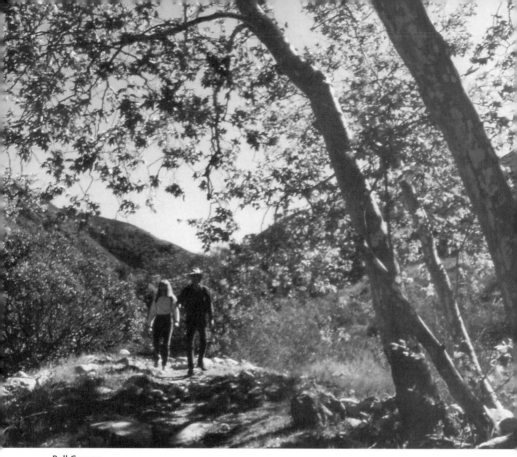

Bell Canyon

Trail. Turn north, skirting the fence line of Rancho Mission Viejo, a vast landholding that encompasses much of southern Orange County and formerly included (before World War II) all of Camp Pendleton as well. To the left and right there are good views of both Bell Canyon and Canada Gobernadora ("Canyon of the Governor's Wife"—though a less literal meaning refers to the invasive chamise, or greasewood, that used to fill the canyon). Canada Gobernadora is now largely given over to agriculture and to the exclusive Coto de Caza housing development, which has spread southward in recent years. The confluence of Canada Gobernadora and San Juan Canyon is one of several supposed sites for Mission Vieja, the original San Juan Capistrano Mission, founded in 1776.

After 0.7 mile on the West Ridge Trail, turn right on Star Rise—the dirt road descending toward Bell Canyon. On the left is a flat terrace, and a resting bench with a commanding view of almost the entire park. You can look down on the line of oaks and sycamores in Bell Canyon below.

At the bottom of the Star Rise downgrade, return toward the starting point using the beautiful Oak Trail and the Nature Trail Loop right near the end.

TRIP 4 East Ridge-Bell Canyon Loop

Distance	6.7 miles, Loop
Hiking Time	3 hours
Elevation Gain/Loss	900'/900'
Difficulty	Moderate
Trail Use	Suitable for mountain biking
Best Times	October through May
Agency	CWP
Optional Map	USGS 7.5-min *Canada Gobernadora*
Notes	Marked trails/obvious routes, easy terrain

DIRECTIONS Exit Interstate 5 at Ortega Highway (Highway 74) in San Juan Capistrano. Proceed east 7.6 miles to Caspers Wilderness Park on the left.

On this hike or ride (mountain bikes are welcome on the specific route described here) you'll pass through two very different kinds of natural habitat: first, a scruffy mix of drought-resistant coastal sage-scrub and chaparral plants on the sunny hillsides and ridges; second, the moisture-loving oak-and-sycamore woodlands along Bell Canyon.

Park you car in one of the lots at the historic windmill/old corral area, and begin the trip by going 0.6 mile south on the paved road. Turn left at East Ridge Trail (a wide fire road). You commence a steady, seldom-steep ascent north along the ridge parallel to and east of Bell Canyon. Dead ahead lies the summit of Santiago Peak, Orange County's high point, some 10 miles north and almost a mile higher.

Aside from the usual California sagebrush, white sage, black sage, and laurel sumac of the sage-scrub community, several common chaparral-community plants make their appearance as you climb: chamise, toyon, yucca, deerweed, manzanita, and elderberry. Here and there you'll pass some dense thickets of prickly pear cactus.

After 2.5 miles of ascent along the east ridge, there's a slightly higher knoll to the east—Pointed Hill. Walk over to it and you'll be treated to a grand view up San Juan Canyon toward the higher Santa Anas.

Back on East Ridge, the trail turns abruptly left and descends a grassy slope to the west. At the bottom, turn right on the Cougar Pass Trail and continue 0.2 mile through a cluster of oaks to the intersection of the Oso Trail, where you turn left toward Bell Canyon. After a little climbing you level off and begin crossing a grassy terrace before dropping again. This flat area is a remnant of one of three or four ancient river terraces exposed on the wall of Bell Canyon. Each terrace represents a stage when Bell Creek became stabilized and used most of its energy to widen its bed rather than cut a deeper channel. Between these quiescent stages, tectonic uplift or other factors, such as a change to a wetter climate, rejuvenated the creek, which then rapidly cut itself to a lower level. Today the creek is engaged in a period of widening, as evidenced by the canyon's broad, flat floor.

Upon reaching the canyon floor, turn left on the Bell Canyon Trail, yet another

Caspers Wilderness Park

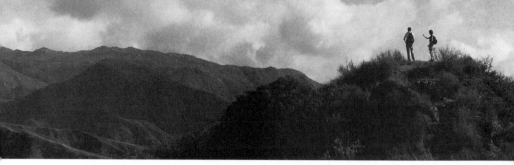

Pointed Hill

fire road, and follow it all the way back (2 more miles) to the old corral and windmill. You won't likely find water tumbling down the bouldery bed of Bell Canyon, unless it's rained a lot recently—though there's plenty underground to support scattered sycamore and oaks.

In the last mile, where the trail gains a little elevation and sticks to the left side of the canyon bottom, you'll find native coast cholla cactus, prickly pear cactus, and various sage-scrub and chaparral plants. Some of the naturalized non-natives include wild oats and rye grass, filaree, mustard, artichoke thistle, milk thistle, and tree tobacco. Here, in the transition zone between the shady woodland along the creek and the warm, dry slopes, your chances of spotting wildlife and birds are greatest. Look for deer, coyotes, bobcats, mountain lions, and a host of smaller creatures. When the ground is wet, tracks easily give away their presence.

TRIP 5 Oso Trail-Juaneno Trail Loop

Distance	9.0 miles, Loop
Hiking Time	5 hours
Elevation Gain/Loss	2200'/2200'
Difficulty	Moderately strenuous
Best Times	November through April
Agency	CWP
Optional Map	USGS 7.5-min *Canada Gobernadora*
Notes	Marked trails/obvious routes, easy terrain

DIRECTIONS   Exit Interstate 5 at Ortega Highway (Highway 74) in San Juan Capistrano. Proceed east 7.6 miles to Caspers Wilderness Park on the left.

Pick a clear, cool day, and set aside the better part of it for this hike to one of the highest ridges in Caspers Wilderness Park. You'll have a wonderful view of the higher Santa Anas, the Los Angeles Basin, the San Joaquin Hills, and the ocean. You'll return along San Juan Creek, meandering in and out of the shade of oaks and sycamores.

Park at the San Juan Meadow group area or at the visitor center, and begin by walking north up the paved road into Bell Canyon. Past the end of the pavement, continue north on the Bell Canyon Trail (dirt road) for one mile, then bear right on the Cougar Pass Trail. Continue northeast another mile on Cougar Pass Trail, up and over a river-terrace remnant, briefly through a cluster of oaks, and to a junction with Oso Trail. Turn right on Oso Trail and follow it straight up the spine of a ridge blanketed with prickly pear cacti. After blooming yellow, orange, or red in the spring and early summer, these cacti grow bulblike fruits, loaded with black seeds, along the edges of their paddle-shaped leaves. The fruits themselves, best displayed in October and November, exhibit a variety of bizarre colors best described as shades of purple, magenta, and red.

Up ahead on the brow of the ridge, a shade ramada with picnic table awaits the footsore. Here you can savor the most panoramic view you're going to get on this hike. The Oso Trail continues farther along the ridgeline, but our way descends south along a crooked firebreak—the Badger Pass Trail—toward San Juan Creek.

When you reach the bottom, next to the Ortega Highway bridge over San Juan Creek, go right on the San Juan Creek Trail. You could follow this highway-paralleling mountain-biking route all the way back, but after just 0.2 mile you have the option of veering right on the narrow and much more interesting Juaneno Trail.

Follow the Juaneno Trail's winding course downstream along the west side of San Juan Creek's usually dry flood plain. Sometimes you're along cobbled banks dotted with riparian vegetation. Other times you swing onto terraces delightfully shaded by oak trees. Bluffs consisting of buff-colored marine sedimentary rock soar dramatically on your right. At one point you circle a covelike indentation in the cliff wall, reminiscent of the stone amphitheaters in Zion National Park.

After a final detour up and over a wooded slope overlooking the flood plain, the trail emerges at the east end of the San Juan Meadow group area, near your starting point.

Oso Trail Vista

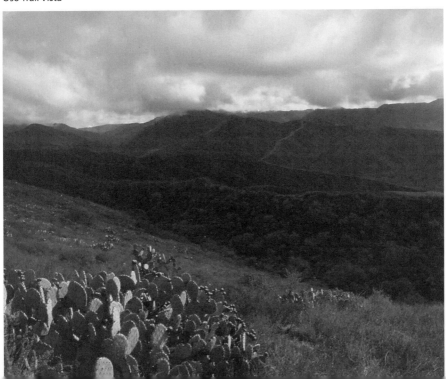

TRIP 6 Cold Spring Canyon Loop

Distance	4.0 miles, Loop
Hiking Time	2½ hours
Elevation Gain/Loss	900'/900'
Difficulty	Moderate
Best Times	October through June
Agency	CWP
Optional Map	USGS 7.5-min *Canada Gobernadora*
Notes	Marked trails/obvious routes, moderate terrain

DIRECTIONS Exit Interstate 5 at Ortega Highway (Highway 74) in San Juan Capistrano. Proceed east 12.5 miles to Hot Springs Canyon Road on the left.

Filled with tall, slender alder trees and spreading oaks, Cold Spring Canyon is one of the most beautiful spots in Caspers Wilderness Park. On a ridge just above Cold Spring Canyon, you'll get a wide-open view of rugged, brush-covered hillsides uncut by roads or trails or any other perceptible form of human alteration as far as the eye can see. Such refreshing vistas are a rare thing to be treasured in today's Orange County.

Assuming you enter at Hot Springs Canyon Road, head west around the remains of the San Juan Hot Springs resort, which welcomed visitors for camping and hot-tubbing until the catastrophic firestorm of October 1993 completely incinerated the place. Follow the San Juan Creek Trail west, paralleling the highway, until you come to Cold Spring Canyon, a deep ravine with a stream flowing through during the wet half of the year.

Unlike the other hikes in Caspers Park, this one begins along Hot Springs Canyon Road on the park's east border, near the San Juan Fire Station. It is important to check the status of this entry, since in recent years a fence has blocked entry into Caspers Park from this direction. You'll need to stop in at the Caspers entrance station to ascertain how to get access to the Cold Spring Canyon loop hike described here.

Pick up the Cold Springs Trail and follow it north up the canyon a short distance. The trail gains a toehold on the slope to the left and soon veers upward along a firebreak. The view keeps expanding as you climb, and soon encompasses the pristine upper reaches of Cold Spring Canyon.

After 500 vertical feet of ascent, you meet the Oso Trail (a fire road). To make this hike a loop trip, stay left and continue west on the Oso Trail, which descends into and then along the bottom of a sunny canyon full of sage-scrub vegetation. That vegetation includes plenty of hardy laurel sumacs, whose leaves remain bright green even through the most intense periods of drought.

At the bottom of the Oso Trail, alongside Ortega Highway, turn left and follow the San Juan Creek Trail back to the starting point. The stretch between Oso Trail and Cold Springs Trail is a bit arduous, as it abruptly climbs high onto the hillside overlooking the highway and later descends.

Chapter 11

Foothills:
Santa Rosa Plateau
Ecological Reserve

The Santa Rosa Plateau, on a southeastern spur of the Santa Ana Mountains, rises over the rapidly expanding suburban communities of southwest Riverside County like a Shangri-La in the sky. In the early 1980s hardly anyone knew of its existence or its ecological significance. Starting with a nucleus of 3100 acres purchased by The Nature Conservancy from a housing-development company in 1983, the current ecological reserve on the plateau now includes more than 8000 acres—some 13 square miles. Today, the reserve is cooperatively managed by The Nature Conservancy and several public agencies. About 40 percent of the reserve is classified as a research area with no public access, about 40 percent is laced with dirt roads and trails for use by hikers only, and the remaining 20 percent or so has "multi-use" roads and trails open to hiking, horseback riding, and mountain biking.

A circle, 100 miles in radius, centered on the reserve, encompasses a megalopolis of some 20 million people. File this fact away in your mind, and then try to fathom its truth while walking amid the green and golden hills of this exquisitely beautiful place. Here is a classic California landscape of wind-rippled grasses, swaying poppies, statuesque oak trees,

Engelmann Oak

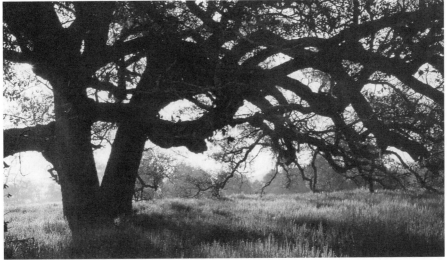

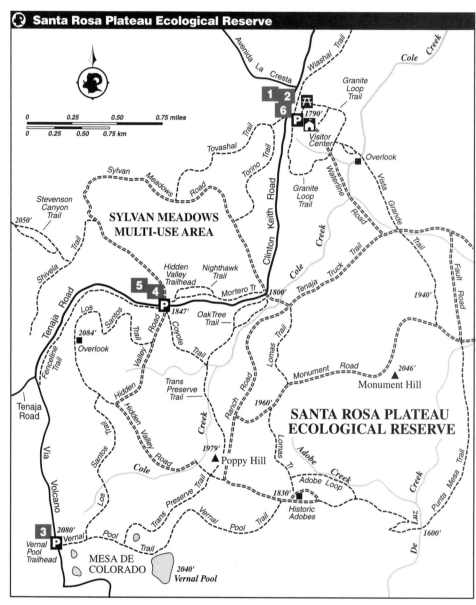

Santa Rosa Plateau Ecological Reserve

trickling streams, vernal pools, and a dazzling assortment of native plants (around 500 at last count) and animals. You will be struck by the reserve's timelessness and insularity, and you will quickly realize how important it was to save it.

Every Southern Californian should have at least one chance to see the Santa Rosa Plateau reserve at its stunning best—during March and April, following a wet winter. The blooming of wildflowers, including California poppies, can be fantastic. Make a note in your calendar now to pay a visit during the next spring season.

TRIP **1** Granite Loop

Distance	1.6 miles, Loop
Hiking Time	1 hour
Elevation Gain/Loss	100'/100'
Difficulty	Easy
Trail Use	Good for kids
Best Times	All year
Agency	SRPER
Optional Map	USGS 7.5-min *Wildomar*
Notes	Marked trails/obvious routes, easy terrain

DIRECTIONS Exit Interstate 15 at Clinton Keith Road in Murrieta (Riverside County). Proceed south on Clinton Keith Road 5 miles to the Santa Rosa Plateau visitor center, on the left.

This mini tour, circling the visitor center, will introduce you to a variety of contrasting habitats within Santa Rosa Plateau Ecological Reserve. The inclusion of a 0.4-mile side trip to and from the east end of the 1.2-mile Granite Loop route lets you visit some tenajas (pools) along Cole Creek and a nice bit of willow and sycamore woodland.

Start the Granite Loop by going north from the west side of the parking lot (don't take the nearby Wiashal Multi-use Trail, which also goes north). Right away, a slight negative change in elevation results in a big change of habitat. You go from sunny chaparral to shadowy live oak woods in only a couple of minutes. Picnic tables are amid the oaks, overlooking a small ravine. The trail continues down along that ravine, then climbs onto a bouldery, chaparral-clad slope on the right.

At 0.4 mile you pass a short-cut trail on the right going back toward the visitor center. At 0.6 mile (right before the Granite Loop trail crosses Waterline Road) you come to the Vista Grande Trail, intersecting on the left. Follow the Vista Grande Trail (out and later back) to visit the

Tenajas Overlook, with a view of Cole Creek. An interpretive panel explains how the tenajas, or small basins worn into the granitic bedrock here are instrumental in supporting the web of life in the reserve during times of drought. In a wet year, the waters of Cole Creek form a large and attractive reflective pool here.

Back on the Granite Loop, cross Waterline Road (dirt road) and enjoy the

Cole Creek from Tenajas Overlook

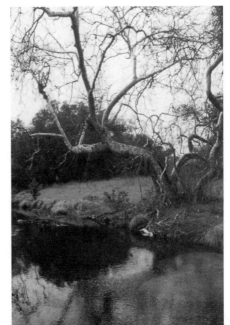

next 0.3 mile in particular as you stroll through a parklike landscape of spreading live oak trees. At two sites, sitting benches are provided under the oldest, most spectacular oaks. Nearing the end of the loop, you climb just a bit and finish the hike amid sunny chaparral.

TRIP 2 Sylvan Meadows

Distance	5.7 miles, Loop
Hiking Time	2½ hours
Elevation Gain/Loss	500'/500'
Difficulty	Moderate
Trail Use	Suitable for mountain biking
Best Times	November through May
Agency	SRPER
Optional Map	USGS 7.5-min *Wildomar*
Notes	Marked trails/obvious routes, easy terrain

DIRECTIONS Exit Interstate 15 at Clinton Keith Road in Murrieta (Riverside County). Proceed south on Clinton Keith Road 5 miles to the Santa Rosa Plateau visitor center, on the left.

The Santa Rosa Plateau's Sylvan Meadows Multi-Use Area is open to all non-motorized means of travel—hiking, jogging, biking, and horseback riding—with the stipulation that all users stay on the designated roads and trails. (Dogs, however, are not allowed here or elsewhere in the reserve.) The comprehensive tour of the whole Sylvan Meadows area, described here, includes an out-and-back side trip into Stevenson Canyon that would seem to be superfluous, but should not be missed.

From the Visitor Center parking lot, cross to the west side of Clinton Keith Road and descend 0.1 mile to a trail junction in a shady ravine. Turn right on the Tovashal Trail (Torino Trail ahead is your return route). After proceeding 0.8 mile up through and eventually out of the shallow ravine, you come to the next junction, Sylvan Meadows Road, on the

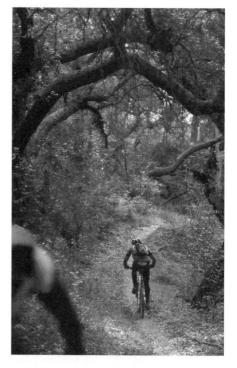

Stevenson Canyon Trail

north edge of an expansive, oak-dotted meadow. This is a part of the roughly 3000 acres of "bunchgrass prairie" in the reserve that is regarded as the finest example of native grassland habitat in California. Ongoing prescribed fires and selective removal of nonnative grasses in meadows such as this one are encouraging the growth of natives such as purple needlegrass, malpais blue grass, and deergrass.

Make a right on Sylvan Meadows Road, continue 0.5 mile along the rim of the meadow, and then begin the highly recommended side trip: Turn right on the Shivela Trail, continue 0.4 mile, then go right again on the Stevenson Canyon Trail. The trail loops, so you can go up along the brushy slope east of the canyon, and back down on a single-track pathway down through the canyon bottom itself. This latter trail segment is arguably the

most enchanting passage in the entire reserve, with inky shadows, a gallery of twisted oak limbs, a trickling stream (in season at least), and luminescent greenery everywhere. Mountain bikers may breeze through here without warning, so those on foot should be alert.

Retrace your steps on Shivela Trail, and then use Sylvan Meadows Road to reach Hidden Valley Trailhead (restrooms are here but no water is available). Now, head east, more or less along the northside fenceline of Tenaja Road, first on Nighthawk Trail and then on Mortero Trail, to the right-angle bend where paved Clinton Keith and Tenaja Roads join. That's where the east leg of Sylvan Meadows Road intersects. It will take you 0.5 mile north to Torino Trail, and Torino Trail will lead you 0.7 mile to the junction you passed at the beginning, just shy of the visitor center.

TRIP 3 Vernal Pool Trail

Distance	1.2 miles round trip, Out-and-back
Hiking Time	1 hour (round trip)
Elevation Gain/Loss	50'/50'
Difficulty	Easy
Trail Use	Good for kids
Best Times	January through May
Agency	SRPER
Optional Map	USGS 7.5-min *Wildomar*
Notes	Marked trails/obvious routes, easy terrain

DIRECTIONS Exit Interstate 15 at Clinton Keith Road in Murrieta (Riverside County). Proceed south on Clinton Keith Road. Note the turnoff for the Santa Rosa Plateau visitor center, 5 miles from I-15. Continue (without making any turns but following the curves of the roadway) to the Vernal Pool trailhead on the left, 3.7 miles from the visitor center.

O ne of the largest vernal pools in California (39 acres at maximum capacity) lies in a shallow depression atop

near-flat Mesa de Colorado on the south side of the Santa Rosa Plateau Ecological Reserve. Getting there is very simple.

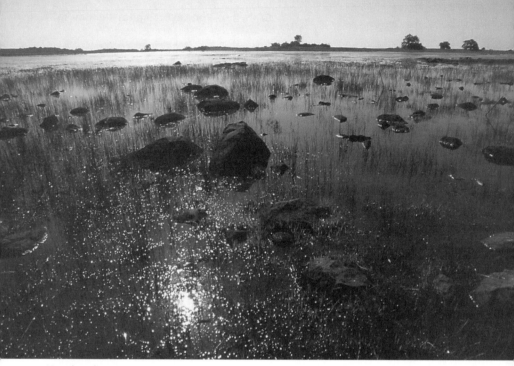

Vernal pool

Drive to the Vernal Pool trailhead, on Via Volcano just 1 mile south of Tenaja Road. Walk due east on the wide, nearly flat Vernal Pool Trail for 0.6 mile to reach the north edge of the large pool, where a boardwalk allows you to approach the "shoreline." On winter and spring weekends, this is far and away the most popular trail in the reserve.

The hard-pan surface underneath vernal pools is generally impervious to water, so once filled during winter storms, the pools dry only by evaporation. Unusual and sometimes unique species of flowering plants have evolved around the perimeter of many vernal pools, including this one. As the pool's perimeter contracts during the steadily lengthening and warming days of spring, successive waves of annual wildflowers bloom along the pool's moist margin. By July or August, there's nothing to be seen but a desiccated depression, its barren surface glaring in the hot sun.

The large pool is also a home for fairy shrimp of several species, and for the spadefoot toad, whose egg clusters may be quite conspicuous.

TRIP 4 Oak Tree Loop

Distance	2.1 miles round trip, Out-and-back
Hiking Time	1 hour (round trip)
Elevation Gain/Loss	100'/100'
Difficulty	Easy
Trail Use	Good for kids
Best Times	All year
Agency	SRPER
Optional Map	USGS 7.5-min *Wildomar*
Notes	Marked trails/obvious routes, easy terrain

DIRECTIONS Exit Interstate 15 at Clinton Keith Road in Murrieta (Riverside County). Proceed south on Clinton Keith Road. Note the turnoff for the Santa Rosa Plateau visitor center, 5 miles from I-15. Continue (without making any turns but following the curves of the roadway) to the Hidden Valley trailhead on the left, 1.5 miles from the visitor center.

The Oak Tree Trail loop takes you through one of the few protected, self-reproducing stands of Engelmann oaks remaining on Earth. The Engelmann oak (or mesa oak), native to the coastal foothills of Southern California and far-northern Baja California, is rapidly being displaced by urbanization and other forms of habitat degradation. These trees are easily distinguishable from their botanical cousins and frequent neighbors—coast live oaks—by their grayish scaly bark (especially on young specimens) and by their grayish-blue-green leaves. Ranging in age up to about 300 years, these particular thick-trunked Engelmanns have real character. Their multifarious, wandering limbs divide into innumerable branches, and their dense foliage spreads outward to cast black pools of shade upon the ground.

There's much more to see along this little trail than just oaks. Cole Creek trickles alongside one leg of the trail, its bed sculpted with small tenajas that support frogs, pond turtles, and newts. California sycamores twine upward among

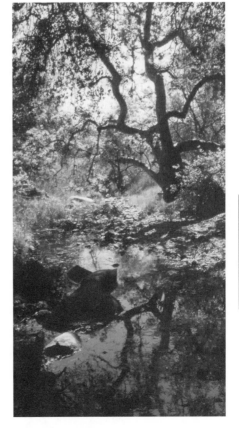

On the Oak Tree Trail

the oaks. One of these oaks has a hollow interior, providing nesting habitat for birds such as woodpeckers and screech owls.

Touring the short (0.6-mile) Oak Tree Trail requires that you hoof it a while before you reach it. From the Hidden Valley Trailhead (on Tenaja Road, 1.7 miles beyond the Visitor Center), walk 0.5 mile southeast on the Coyote Trail, and then make a left on the Trans Preserve Trail to connect with the Oak Tree loop. Along the way, over gently rolling, grassy terrain, take note of purple needlegrass—a native, fire-resistant and drought-resistant bunchgrass that survives by sending down roots several feet deep. The landscape here, partially restored by techniques such as prescribed burning, is a rare facsimilie of what much of coastal Southern California looked like centuries ago.

After you've walked fully around the Oak Tree Loop, retrace your footsteps on the Trans Preserve and Coyote trails.

TRIP 5 Los Santos-Trans Preserve Loop

Distance	4.8 miles, Loop
Hiking Time	2½ hours
Elevation Gain/Loss	500'/500'
Difficulty	Moderate
Best Times	November through May
Agency	SRPER
Optional Map	USGS 7.5-min *Wildomar*
Notes	Marked trails/obvious routes, easy terrain

DIRECTIONS Exit Interstate 15 at Clinton Keith Road in Murrieta (Riverside County). Proceed south on Clinton Keith Road. Note the turnoff for the Santa Rosa Plateau visitor center, 5 miles from I-15. Continue (without making any turns but following the curves of the roadway) to the Hidden Valley trailhead on the left, 1.5 miles from the visitor center.

This loop hike traverses the open meadows, grassy hillsides, and shady recesses of the reserve's southwest corner. You'll enjoy superb views throughout, plus excellent opportunities for bird and wildlife watching.

Begin at Hidden Valley Trailhead by heading uphill (south) on the wide Hidden Valley Road. After only 0.2 mile, make a right on the narrow Los Santos Trail. This delightfully primitive path crookedly ascends some bald hillsides, gains a ridgetop, and passes a resting bench just south of a 2084-foot knoll. From this overlook point, the bulk of the reserve's sensuously rolling terrain lies in full view. Perhaps this is the ideal spot to break out your high-powered binoculars to scan for deer in the meadows below and to track raptors gliding in the sky above.

Beyond the overlook, the Los Santos Trail drops into an upper tributary of Cole Creek and bends left to follow the tributary's tiny (and usually dry) brook. After just 0.1 mile, the path ahead assumes the proportions of a dirt road and continues southeast to join Hidden Valley Road. Don't miss the sign on the right, which directs you onto the sharply ascending, again delightfully primitive, south branch of the Los Santos Trail.

You climb to the lip of an oak-dotted plateau, a northward extension of the nearby Mesa de Colorado. Underfoot, there are small outcrops of basalt, a dark-colored volcanic rock. Basalt underlies the entire plateau, and its tough, erosion-resistant character is responsible for the plateau's elevated position. The softer, marine sedimentary rocks associated with the terrain behind you have eroded to form all those sensuously rolling hills and valleys.

In spring, look for the dark brown blossoms of chocolate lilies, coyly exposing themselves under the semi-shade of the oaks.

Los Santos Trail continues south, dipping into and out of a shady ravine, then enters Mesa de Colorado proper, where you arrive at a junction with the Vernal Pool Trail. You've now come 2.4 miles, exactly half way around the loop.

Turn left on the Vernal Pool Trail, proceed 0.3 mile, and turn left on the Trans Preserve Trail. (Note: the large vernal pool lies just ahead on the Vernal Pool Trail; don't miss it, especially if you haven't seen it before.)

On the Trans Preserve Trail, you meander northeast, descend off the plateau rim by way of an oblique course down a gorgeously oak-draped hillside, and strike a near-level, northward course alongside Poppy Hill—one of several good sites in the reserve for viewing California poppies in the springtime. On ahead, you gently curve and descend along another Cole Creek tributary ravine, and (4.3 miles into the hike) you reach the Coyote Trail. Turn left and complete the remaining half mile to Hidden Valley Trailhead.

Trans Preserve Trail

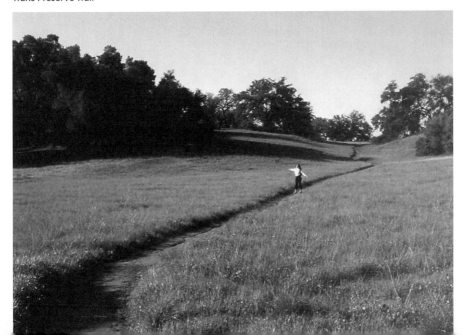

TRIP 6 Punta Mesa Loop

Distance	8.0 miles, Loop
Hiking Time	4 hours
Elevation Gain/Loss	650'/650'
Difficulty	Moderately strenuous
Best Times	December through May
Agency	SRPER
Optional Map	USGS 7.5-min *Wildomar*
Notes	Marked trails/obvious routes, easy terrain

DIRECTIONS Exit Interstate 15 at Clinton Keith Road in Murrieta (Riverside County). Proceed south on Clinton Keith Road 5 miles to the Santa Rosa Plateau visitor center, on the left.

For a comprehensive tour of the Santa Rosa Plateau Ecological Reserve, try this half-day hike, which will introduce you to virtually every attractive feature characteristic of Southern California's foothills. The hike is probably far too hot and dry for most people during the warmer half of the year, but it's pleasant during the winter and on cool springtime days.

Start your journey at the Visitor Center. Follow the dirt road going southeast—Waterline Road. At 0.8 mile, turn right on Teneja Truck Trail and traverse its flat, straight course across a treeless plain. At 1.7 miles, near the junction of Ranch Road, make a left on the narrow Lomas Trail. Ascend a slope dotted with Engelmann oaks, jog right for about 0.2 mile on Monument Road, and then find the continuation of Lomas Trail on the left. You now make a descent into a valley, where the Adobe Loop trail branches left, and two adobe buildings set amid towering oaks lie just ahead. Those are the adobes of the former Santa Rosa Ranch, and you won't want to miss visiting them. Constructed around 1845, they are Riverside County's oldest standing structures. Your hike has taken you 3 miles so far.

After a look at the adobes and a refreshing pause in the shade, backtrack 0.1 mile north on Lomas Trail and take the Adobe Loop trail east, down along an oak-filled canyon. Enjoy the last deeply shaded stretch of trail you're going to get on this hike. Soon enough, it's back into

Veranda of the Old Adobe

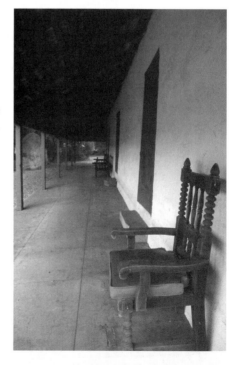

the sunshine again as you climb up to a junction with the Punta Mesa Trail. Turn left and follow this deteriorating former fire road a total of 2 miles—down across De Luz Creek and back uphill, heading north. Mesa de la Punta, rising to the south and Mesa de Burro to the east, both capped with erosion-resistant basalt, are part of the reserve's off-limits-to-the-public research zone.

At the next intersection (a total of 5.8 miles into the hike), turn left on Monument Road, travel 0.2 mile west, and veer right on the aptly named Vista Grande Trail. Follow Vista Grande Trail north to a crest (elevation 1940′), where your gaze takes in hundreds of acres of wind-rippled grass and the distant, winter-snow-capped San Bernardino and San Jacinto mountains. Curving northwest, the Vista Grande Trail crosses Tenaja Truck Trail and then more or less makes a beeline for the visitor center, traversing near-flat ter-

rain punctuated with scattered oaks and lichen-encrusted piles of granitic rock.

Vista Grande Trail

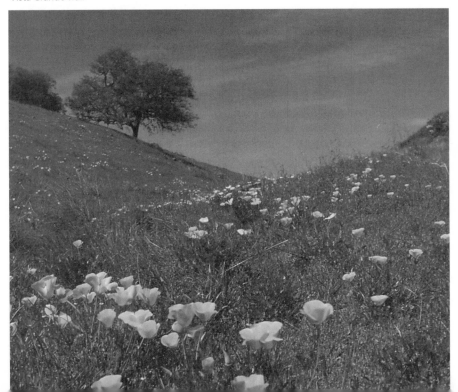

Chapter 12

Santa Ana Mountains— Main Divide

Most of the higher Santa Ana Mountains—along with their extensions to the southeast and east—the Elsinore and Santa Margarita mountains, lie within the overall boundary of Cleveland National Forest, fixed by Congress in 1908. Today the administrative subunit covering this area is called the Trabuco Ranger District. Of the 255 square miles encompassed by the district, about 210 square miles are managed by the federal government. Private "inholdings" make up the difference.

In this book we divide the Trabuco District into three parts—northern, middle, and southern—because of the distinctly different character of each one. In this section, covering most of what is called the "Main Divide" of the Santa Ana Mountains, visitor facilities are almost nil, but an extensive dirt-road system, along with a few trails, makes it relatively easy for hikers to get around. The middle section (Chapter 13) along Ortega Highway has camping facilities, many trails, and good access to them. The southern section (Chapter 14), San Mateo Canyon Wilderness, has an extensive trail system that receives varying degrees of maintenance.

Geographically, the Main Divide is an important watershed divide, featuring several of the Santa Ana's highest peaks.

These include (from north to south) Sierra Peak; Pleasants Peak; Bedford Peak; Bald Peak; Modjeska and Santiago peaks, together forming the familiar "Old Saddleback"; and Trabuco Peak. These rounded summits (except Modjeska) serve, in connect-the-dots fashion, as benchmarks for the Orange/Riverside county line.

East of the Main Divide, water flows down steep-cut canyons to Temescal Valley—a shallow depression on the far side of the Elsinore Fault—where it usually percolates into the water table. During times of exceptional flood the runoff may make its way north to Corona and the Santa Ana River.

West of the divide, water flows down canyons steep in their upper reaches, narrow and rather straight in their midsections, and broad and gently meandering through the foothills. If not claimed by percolation or detained by dams, the water makes its way across Orange County's coastal plain—typically in concrete-lined channels—to the sea.

The Main Divide appears treeless and rather austere from a distance, yet it holds many surprises. The ubiquitous chaparral and sage-scrub cover that appears half-dead in summer's blazing heat turns bright green and pleasingly pungent at the touch of late autumn's first steady rain. Early spring sunshine brings forth a profusion of blossoms and perfumelike aromas.

On both sides of the Main Divide, coniferous trees cling to moist pockets of soil, and scattered springs feed perennial and seasonal creeks that in turn sustain willows, sycamores, maples, bay laurels, and centuries-old oaks in the bottoms of the deepest ravines and canyons.

Much of the serenity and ecological integrity of the north Santa Ana Mountains could be sacrificed if a proposed freeway link between Interstate 15 at Cajalco Road in Riverside County and the Eastern Transportation Corridor toll road in Orange County ever becomes a reality. Considerable debate is likely to take place on this issue in the coming years.

Inside Coal Canyon

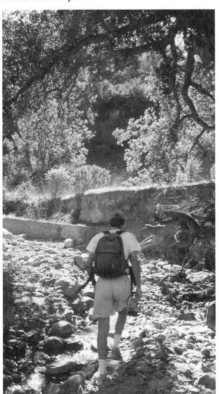

The Main Divide's existing road system, which consists largely of unpaved roads, serves purposes as diverse as fire control, access to utility and telecommunications facilities, recreational driving, hiking, and mountain biking. In the recent past, these roads have been closed to vehicles—part time or all the time—for reasons such as storm damage, fire danger, and the protection of endangered species such as the arroyo toad. For the latest information on road closures for vehicles in the Santa Ana Mountains, call the Trabuco Ranger District office in Corona (951-736-1811), or visit www.fs.fed.us/r5/cleveland, and look at the web page titled "Current Conditions."

Hikers and mountain bikers usually have the privilege of unrestricted travel on the Main Divide's roads and trails, but not when the Forest Service declares an emergency fire closure during extremely dry weather, or when an order is issued to protect endangered species. Again, by phone or internet, you may find out the latest information from the forest service.

At all times and in all seasons "no fires/no camping" is the unbending rule in the Main Divide area—though hiking before dawn and after sunset is not prohibited.

Most of the trailheads for the trips below lie on national forest land and therefore are subject to the "National Forest Adventure Pass" program. The rules are constantly in a state of flux—but basically, visitors must purchase an adventure pass (parking permit) for the privilege of parking their cars along roadsides, in picnic grounds, or at trailheads in any national forest in Southern California. The permit, which costs $5 daily or $30 yearly, can be purchased at any national forest office or ranger station, and at virtually every Southern California outdoor equipment and sports vendor.

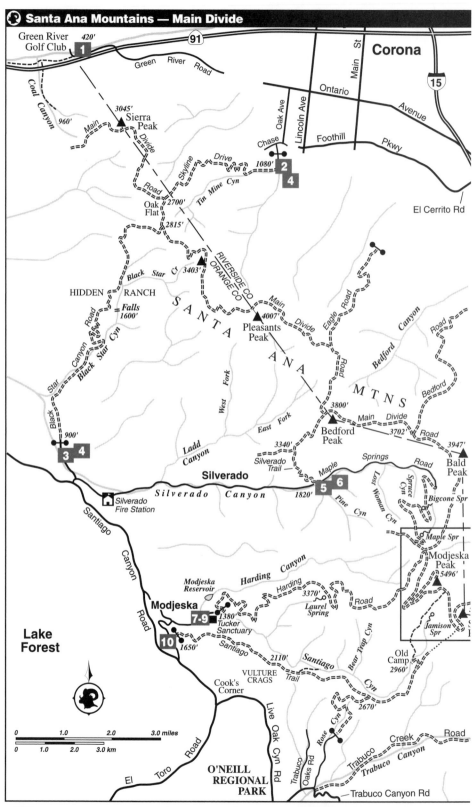

Green River
Golf Club *420'*
1

91

Green River Road

Coal Canyon
960'

Main Divide

3045'
Sierra
Peak

Skyline Drive

Tin Mine Cyn

1080'
2
4

Chase

Corona

Main St

Oak Ave

Lincoln Ave

Ontario

Foothill

Avenue

15

Pkwy

El Cerrito Rd

Oak
Flat
2700'

2815'

Black Star Cr *3403'*

HIDDEN RANCH

*Falls
1600'*

Black Star Cyn

Black Star Canyon Road

S A N T A

RIVERSIDE CO
ORANGE CO

Pleasants
Peak
4007'

Main Divide

Eagle Road

Bedford Canyon Road

A N A

M T N S

Bedford

West Fork

East Fork

3800'
Bedford
Peak

Main Divide
3702'
Road

3947'
Bald
Peak

900'
3 **4**

Ladd
Canyon

3340'
Silverado Trail

Silverado

Maple Springs Road

Spruce Cyn

Low Woman Cyn

Bigcone Spr

🏠 Silverado
Fire Station

Silverado Canyon
1820'
5 **6**

Pine Cyn

Maple Spr

Santiago

Canyon Road

**Lake
Forest**

Modjeska
Reservoir

Harding Canyon

Harding
3370'
Road

Laurel
Spring

Modjeska
Peak
5496'

Jamison
Spr

Modjeska
7-9
1380'
Tucker
Sanctuary

10 *1650'*

Santiago

2110'

Santiago Trail

VULTURE
CRAGS

Cook's
Corner

Bear Trap Cyn

2670'

Old
Camp
2960'

0   1.0   2.0   3.0 miles
0 1.0 2.0 3.0 km

Live Oak Cyn Rd

El Toro Road

**O'NEILL
REGIONAL
PARK**

Rose Cyn

Trabuco Oaks Rd

Trabuco

Creek Road

Trabuco Canyon

Trabuco Canyon Rd

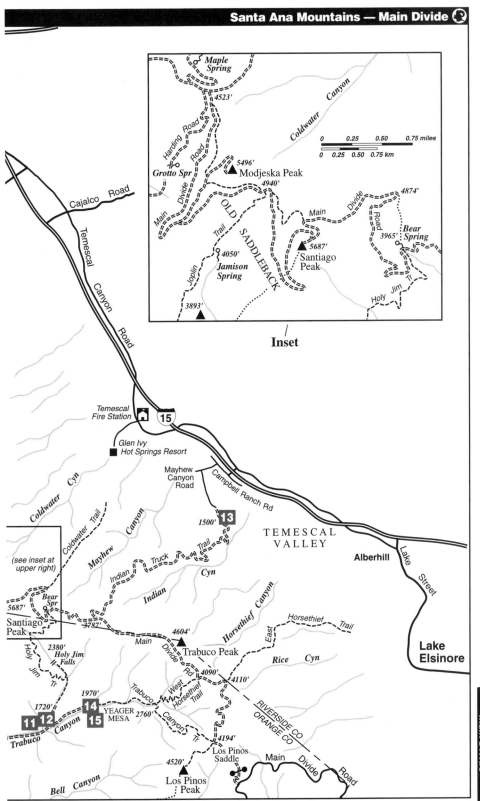

Maple Spring

4523'

Coldwater Canyon

Harding Road

Road

Grotto Spr

| 0 | 0.25 | 0.50 | 0.75 miles |

| 0 | 0.25 | 0.50 | 0.75 km |

5496'

▲ Modjeska Peak

4940'

Main Divide

Main Divide Road

4874'

Trail

Joplin

4050'
Jamison Spring

5687'
▲ Santiago Peak

3965' ○ *Bear Spring*

OLD SADDLEBACK

3893'
▲

Holy Jim Tr

Inset

Cajalco Road

Temescal Canyon Road

Temescal Fire Station

15

Glen Ivy Hot Springs Resort

Mayhew Canyon Road

Campbell Ranch Rd

1500' **13**

T E M E S C A L
V A L L E Y

Alberhill

Coldwater Cyn

Coldwater Trail

Mayhew Canyon

Indian

Truck

Cyn

Indian

(see inset at upper right)

Bear Spr

5687'
Santiago Peak

3782'

2380'
Holy Jim Falls

Holy Jim Tr

Main

4604'
▲ Trabuco Peak

Horsethief Canyon

East

Horsethief *Trail*

Rice Cyn

Lake Elsinore

Lake Street

4090'

4110'

1970'

1720'

Trabuco

14
YEAGER MESA

15

11 **12**

2760'

Canyon

West Horsethief Trail

Tr

RIVERSIDE CO
ORANGE CO

4194'

4520'
▲ Los Pinos Peak

Los Pinos Saddle

Main Divide Road

Bell Canyon

Trabuco

TRIP 1 Coal Canyon

Distance	5.4 miles round trip, Out-and-back
Hiking Time	3 hours (round trip)
Elevation Gain/Loss	600'/600'
Difficulty	Moderate
Best Times	December through April
Agency	CHSP
Optional Map	USGS 7.5-min *Black Star Canyon*
Notes	Marked trails/obvious routes, easy terrain

DIRECTIONS Exit the Riverside Freeway (Highway 91) at Green River Road in Corona, and turn west. After 1 mile, park on the right side of Green River Road where space is available at a point 0.2 mile short of the entrance to the Green River Golf Club.

For at least three decades, the Coal Canyon diamond interchange on the Riverside Freeway through Santa Ana Canyon was a virtual joke, featuring ramps to and from nowhere. "Nowhere" might have been replaced by subdivisions spreading eastward from Yorba Linda and Anaheim Hills. That hasn't happened, and likely will never happen. The Coal Canyon undercrossing, it was discovered, was the one and only practical wildlife corridor between 40,000 acres of undeveloped lands in the Chino and Puente hills to the north and half a million acres of wild land in the Santa Ana Mountains to the south. Mountain lions were using it to avoid being flattened by an endless river of cars, 10 to 12 lanes wide. Biologists increasingly insist that preserving habitat linkages, even lowly ones such as freeway crossings and tunnels, are essential to the regional survival of migratory wild animals.

Coal Canyon's freeway ramps were closed in 2003. The asphalt strip of the putative parkway underneath is gone, and a wide stretch of Coal Canyon south of the freeway is now friendlier to both migrating creatures and hikers curious enough to visit. Formerly under private ownership, the canyon has fallen under the jurisdiction of Chino Hills State Park and California's Department of Fish and Game.

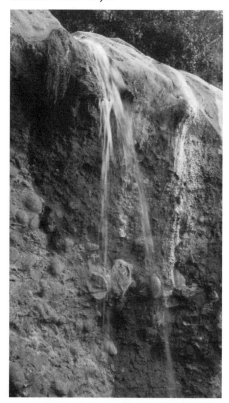
Waterfall in Coal Canyon

From the parking space on Green River Road, walk the 0.2-mile stretch toward the golf course entrance, and continue on the paved Santa Ana River bike trail that closely parallels the freeway. Endure for the next few minutes the insanely roaring traffic on your left. The wide Santa Ana River concrete flood channel lies on your right, and beyond that, the green spaces of the golf course.

When you reach the Coal Canyon crossing after 1.2 miles, walk underneath the overpasses and continue south into Chino Hills State Park territory (signs say no bikes and no dogs allowed). Follow an old, often eroded truck trail up Coal Canyon's wide floodplain, staying to the

left of the canyon's sand-and-gravel-coated stream bed.

After a mile of uphill hiking, just short of where the canyon significantly narrows, you'll need to drop down onto the gravelly canyon floor itself. Proceed 0.5 mile farther upstream, following a silvery strand of water (if there is any), to where the canyon walls soar and pinch in tightly. There—in the wettest time of a wet year—the sound of spattering water heralds your arrival at a sublime grotto graced with a 20-foot high shower of crystal-clear water. It pours off a mineralized outcrop shaped like the spout of a teapot. This is a rare sight in a location that would seem unlikely for a waterfall.

TRIP 2 Sierra Peak via Skyline Drive

Distance	14.5 miles round trip, Out-and-back
Hiking Time	7½ hours (round trip)
Elevation Gain/Loss	3200'/3200'
Difficulty	Strenuous
Trail Use	Dogs allowed, suitable for mountain biking
Best Times	November through March
Agency	CNF/TD
Recommended Map	Cleveland National Forest recreation map
Optional Maps	USGS 7.5-min *Corona South, Black Star Canyon*
Notes	Marked trails/obvious routes, easy terrain

DIRECTIONS Exit the Riverside Freeway (Highway 91) at Lincoln Avenue, and follow Lincoln Avenue 1.7 miles south to Ontario Avenue. Go west on Ontario Avenue 0.3 mile to Oak Avenue, and go south on Oak Avenue for 0.9 mile to Chase Drive. Follow Chase Drive west for 0.2 mile to a narrow road going south—the unsigned Skyline Drive. Park where you can short of the forest gate.

Wait for a winter storm to clear the air, then try this viewful hike to Sierra Peak, the rounded promontory anchoring the north end of the Santa Ana Mountains. Because the route follows well-graded service roads throughout

and the climbing is quite gradual, this is an ideal route for energetic runners and mountain bicyclists as well as hikers.

Around the winter solstice, an afternoon/evening trek to and from Sierra Peak can be very rewarding. Plan to reach the peak in time to watch the sun drop into the Pacific (before 5 P.M. from early November to early January). Then stroll back down under the stars, arriving at your car before 8 P.M. Nights lit by a full or nearly full moon are best; otherwise the glare of the city lights below makes it hard to see the ground underfoot. Don't forget extra warm clothes and a flashlight.

Geologically, this is an interesting area. About 2 miles up from the trailhead, you'll cross the Elsinore Fault zone, with crumbly 150-million-year-old metavolcanic rock to the southwest and colorfully banded marine sedimentary rocks half that age to the northeast. Near Sierra Peak are some nice exposures of sandstone with embedded cobbles.

Begin hiking (or mountain biking) on the dirt road ahead, which is called "Skyline Drive." After the first mile, the road swings back away and up from the mouth of Tin Mine Canyon. A side trail on the left goes a way up the canyon itself. Years ago, the canyon was a designated target-shooting area. Now it's mercifully quiet.

As you curl upward along the ridge north of Tin Mine Canyon, views open up of nearby Corona and the more distant cities of Riverside and San Bernardino, backed up by the towering summits of the San Gabriel and San Bernardino mountains. Some orange groves remain in view, but new subdivisions are replacing them—a symptom of the phenomenal growth of the region known as the Inland Empire.

Oak Flat, 4.8 miles from the gate, is marked by grassland dotted with a few oaks and a radio communications complex. At the road junction turn right (Black Star Canyon Road goes left, south) and continue along the main divide of the Santa Anas toward Sierra Peak, the antenna-bristling summit to the north.

On top there's a great view of the Chino Hills and Pomona Valley to the north, the broad trough of lower Santa Ana Canyon to the west, and endless miles of L.A. Basin suburbia stretching toward the Pacific Ocean.

TRIP 3 Black Star Canyon Falls

Distance	6.6 miles round trip, Out-and-back
Hiking Time	5 hours (round trip)
Elevation Gain/Loss	800'/800'
Difficulty	Moderately strenuous
Best Times	November through May
Agency	CNF/TD
Recommended Map	USGS 7.5-min *Black Star Canyon*
Optional Map	Cleveland National Forest recreation map
Notes	Navigation required, bushwhacking, difficult terrain

DIRECTIONS Exit from either eastern toll road (Highway 241 or 261) at Santiago Canyon Road. Drive 6 miles east to Silverado Canyon Road, turn left, proceed 0.1 mile, and turn left on Black Star Canyon Road. Go 1.1 mile to the forest gate and park.

Good timing is the key to catching the waterfall in Black Star Canyon at its best. Since only about 3 square miles of drainage area lie above it, persistent rains are needed to get more than a dribble of water over the fall. Whether the water is flowing or not, though, the canyon bottom itself is delightful to explore any time the weather is mild.

After an uninteresting half mile along the dry, open bed of Santiago Creek, the road abruptly turns east into Black Star Canyon. Scattered oaks, sycamores, and willows, and rows of planted eucalyptus trees provide shade as the road meanders gently uphill along the creekbed. The canyon was named after the nearby Black Star Coal Mine (on private land), which was worked briefly more than a century ago during a silver- and coal-mining boom in the Silverado Canyon area. Look for seams of poor-quality coal in the roadcuts you pass.

At 2.5 miles the road doubles back in a hairpin turn to ascend the sage-covered slopes to the north. You've now reached the corner of Section 30, which is part of Cleveland National Forest. It's time to put on long pants and a long-sleeved shirt to

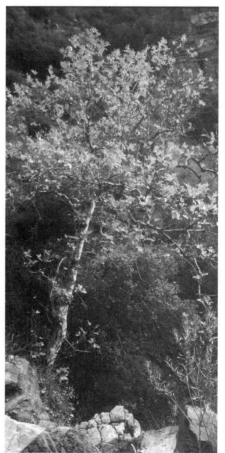

Sycamore in autumn, Black Star Canyon

do battle with poison oak and other shrubbery up the canyon. At least 1 hour (0.8 mile) of boulder-hopping, bush-whacking, and moderate hands-and-feet scrambling up the trenchlike confines of the canyon will take you to the base of the falls.

Marine sedimentary rocks are in evidence here. Bold outcrops of stratified, buff-colored siltstone rise hundreds of feet above the canyon bottom, giving safe quarter to nesting raptors and other birds. The creek slides around great blocks of conglomerate rock and pools up in shady grottos concealed amid large oak, alder, sycamore, and bay trees.

The semicircular siltstone headwall that forms the falls fairly drips with mosses and maidenhair ferns, if not water. When the flow is great enough, water cascades 50 feet down a polished chute, and also exits through an old mine shaft cut into the headwall about 15 feet above the falls' base.

By backtracking down-canyon about 200 yards, and then thrashing up a steep ravine to the west (thus outflanking some crumbling cliffs), it's possible to reach nearby Black Star Canyon Road at the 1960-foot contour. But it's far easier and safer to return the way you came, making your way down the creekbed over now-familiar obstacles.

TRIP 4 North Main Divide Traverse

Distance	13.0 miles, Point-to-point
Hiking Time	6½ hours
Elevation Gain/Loss	1950'/2150'
Difficulty	Moderately strenuous
Trail Use	Dogs allowed, suitable for mountain biking
Best Times	November through April
Agency	CNF/TD
Recommended Maps	USGS 7.5-min *Corona South, Black Star Canyon*; Cleveland National Forest recreation map
Notes	Marked trails/obvious routes, easy terrain

DIRECTIONS NORTH END: Exit the Riverside Freeway (Highway 91) at Lincoln Avenue, and follow Lincoln Avenue 1.7 miles south to Ontario Avenue. Go west on Ontario Avenue 0.3 mile to Oak Avenue, and go south on Oak Avenue for 0.9 mile to Chase Drive. Follow Chase Drive west for 0.2 mile to a narrow road going south—the unsigned Skyline Drive. SOUTH END: Exit from either eastern toll road (Highway 241 or 261) at Santiago Canyon Road. Drive 6 miles east to Silverado Canyon Road, turn left, proceed 0.1 mile, and turn left on Black Star Canyon Road. Go 1.1 mile to the forest gate.

Incorporating parts of Trips 2 and 3 above, this trek over the north crest of the Santa Ana Mountains is perfect for in-shape runners, walkers, and mountain bikers. Relatively easy grades, generally smooth dirt and gravel surfaces, and little or no interference from motor vehicles are yours all the way—though the 13-mile distance is far from trivial. The aftermath of heavy rains, however, can prove to be a serious hindrance especially for cyclists. This is no problem on the Skyline Drive side, but Black Star Canyon Road in the vicinity of Hidden Ranch can turn into one big mudhole.

Because of elevation differences, it's a little easier to begin on the east near Corona and end by way of Black Star Canyon in Orange County. After taking care of transportation arrangements, proceed up the moderate but steady incline of Skyline Drive, starting from that road's vehicle gate in Corona.

Only one brief downhill stretch, about 0.3 mile long, interrupts the climb from the gate to Oak Flat. As you cross the county line just before reaching Oak Flat, you'll spot the first of the many "Black

Star Canyon Road—use at your own risk" signs posted by Orange County.

At 4.8 miles (Oak Flat intersection) turn left (south) and continue uphill toward the next junction, 5.3 miles, where the Main Divide Road forks left. The tumbledown rock houses nearby, labeled "Beeks Place" on the topo map, are surrounded by an unkempt but still-thriving grove of planted trees—natives like Coulter pine, knobcone pine, and Tecate cypress, plus some nonnatives. Not much shade can be found ahead until you reach scattered oaks and sycamores at Hidden Ranch.

From Beeks Place bear right on Black Star Canyon Road and begin the long, winding descent into the grassy bowl occupied by Hidden Ranch. This former privately owned cattle ranch—now a conservancy area and therefore protected

Hidden Valley

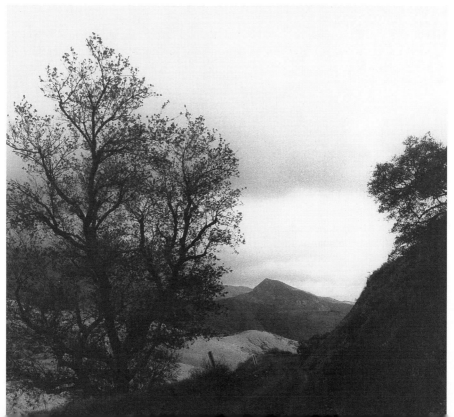

from possible future development—is truly hidden from the sights and sounds of the city below. Hidden Ranch is renowned for its human history. Bedrock mortars here tell of its use as a major Indian village. It was also the site of an 1831 raid on Indian horse thieves, and the site of a notorious murder incident in 1899.

Past Hidden Ranch, Black Star Canyon Road continues its leisurely descent down some sun-blasted, sage-covered slopes. At 8.7 miles the road swings close to the gorge concealing Black Star Canyon falls. Finally, at 10.5 miles, you reach the cool bottom of Black Star Canyon, and the remaining miles to the Black Star Canyon Road vehicle gate are pleasantly shaded.

TRIP 5 Silverado Trail to Bedford Peak

Distance	6.6 miles round trip, Out-and-back
Hiking Time	4 hours (round trip)
Elevation Gain/Loss	2200'/2200'
Difficulty	Moderately strenuous
Trail Use	Dogs allowed
Best Times	October through May
Agency	CNF/TD
Recommended Maps	USGS 7.5-min *Santiago Peak, Corona South;* or Cleveland National Forest recreation map
Notes	Marked trails/obvious routes, easy terrain

DIRECTIONS Exit from either eastern toll road (Highway 241 or 261) at Santiago Canyon Road. Drive 6 miles east to Silverado Canyon Road, and turn left (east). Proceed 5.4 miles to the forest gate (which may or may not be closed to motor traffic) at the east end of the community of Silverado.

This no-nonsense climb to one of the principal summits of the Main Divide is physically demanding enough to serve as an excellent conditioning hike, and scenically rewarding as well. From the Main Divide's west-side trailheads there's no faster way to reach the crest by foot.

On foot now, continue up-canyon past the vehicle gate, which may or may not be closed and locked to keep out vehicles. In about 300 yards, just after crossing the alder-shaded bottom of the canyon, turn sharply to the left (west) on the old roadbed that climbs sharply up the north wall of the canyon. This is the

Silverado Trail (Silverado Motorway on older maps), built originally for fire control, then used for a while by 4-wheel-drive enthusiasts. It is now severely eroded, but suitable enough for hiking.

An excellent view of the whole of Silverado Canyon unfolds as you swing around several hairpin turns. In the road cuts, a well-stratified, often sharply folded metasedimentary rock (the Bedford Canyon Formation) is exposed. The sediments making up these rocks were deposited on the sea floor more than 150 million years ago, buried and metamorphosed by heat and pressure, and finally

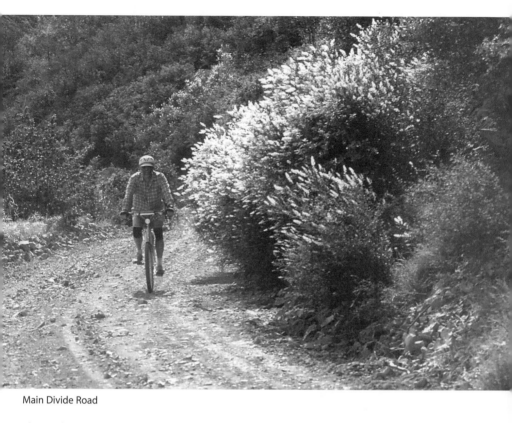

Main Divide Road

elevated to their present position high above sea level.

The trail remains in primitive shape until you reach the shoulder of a ridge overlooking Ladd Canyon to the northwest. You bend to the right, staying on top of that ridge on a graded road striking northeast, toward the Main Divide.

On reaching Main Divide Road (2.9 miles from the start), turn right, continue 0.3 mile, then walk up the rounded 3800-foot summit of Bedford Peak on the right. There's no place to rest comfortably on the open summit, but the view—from the Pacific coast to the peaks of the Peninsular Ranges—can be stupendous on a clear day.

TRIP 6 Silverado-Modjeska Peak Loop

Distance	18.3 miles (to Modjeska Peak and back), Loop
Hiking Time	9 hours
Elevation Gain/Loss	4440'/4440'
Difficulty	Strenuous
Trail Use	Dogs allowed, suitable for mountain biking
Best Times	November through May
Agency	CNF/TD
Recommended Maps	USGS 7.5-min *Santiago Peak, Corona South;* or Cleveland National Forest recreation map
Notes	Marked trails/obvious routes, easy terrain

DIRECTIONS Exit from either eastern toll road (Highway 241 or 261) at Santiago Canyon Road. Drive 6 miles east to Silverado Canyon Road, and turn left (east). Proceed 5.4 miles to the forest gate (which may or may not be closed to motor traffic) at the east end of the community of Silverado.

The goal of this hike, looping up and over the Main Divide, is to reach the summit of Modjeska Peak—the lower, north summit of Old Saddleback. If you omit the out-and-back leg to the peak itself, however, you shorten the trip by 2.5 miles. Either way, this is an all-day trek on foot. During the clear, crisp weather characteristic of certain periods from November through March (and assuming you won't be sharing the roads with any vehicles), this hike can be among the most rewarding and peaceful in Southern California.

Climb to Main Divide Road via Silverado Trail. Turn south past Bedford Peak and follow Main Divide Road for several undulating miles, passing several small summits along the way. Just north of Bald Peak, a big powerline barely clears the ridge. This 500-kilovolt line, completed in 1987, links the Palm Springs area and Orange County.

There are clear lines of sight in most directions, and most of Southern California's highest mountain ranges are in view. Below and to the west, a scant mile away,

you can trace the zigzag path of the Maple Springs Road (your return route) across a sparsely timbered slope and down to the bottom of upper Silverado Canyon.

After 8.7 miles (from the start) Main Divide Road comes to an intersection north of, and about 1000 vertical feet below, imposing Modjeska Peak. Swing left, staying on Main Divide Road, and continue 75 yards. Then, turn onto the obscure trail that angles steeply up the road cut on the left, and continue climbing across a slope. After a half mile, you plunge into the shade of some tall chaparral shrubs and small oak trees. After another 0.3 mile you reach the access road leading to Modjeska Peak. Go left and continue 0.5 mile to Modjeska's open summit. On a clear day, the 360-degree view of the surrounding mountains, basins, and ocean is obstructed only slightly by the antenna-bristling summit of Santiago Peak, a mile southeast. (Note: mountain bikers headed to Modjeska Peak might want to avoid the trail shortcut to the peak and instead go the long

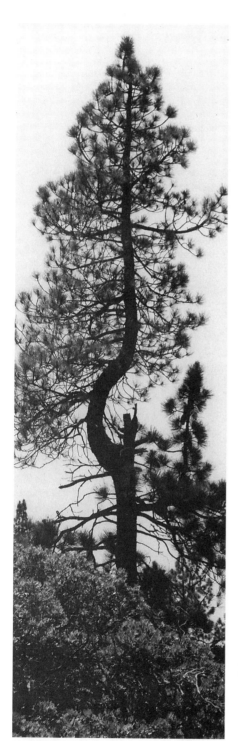

way around using the gradually ascending Main Divide Road.)

Your return to the starting point is now entirely downhill. Retrace your steps to Main Divide Road and continue north to the next road intersection (4523′), and turn left on Maple Springs Road. As you start down, keep right at the next two road intersections so as to stay on Maple Springs Road.

The next several miles on Maple Springs Road are a botanist's delight. On the upper slopes huge Coulter pines soar above thick carpets of manzanita shrubs. Big-cone Douglas-fir, bigleaf maple, bay, and live oak trees crowd together in the larger ravines, casting dense pools of shade over trickling streams.

On the sixth sharp hairpin turn from the top, 4 miles down from Main Divide Road, you finally reach the bottom of Silverado Canyon. Maple Springs Road becomes paved at this point. During the last 3 miles, the stream flows merrily along next to the road, flanked by sycamores, alders, and more maples. In spring, California poppy and golden yarrow brighten the roadside, while the celebrated snowy-white Matilija poppy, the "queen of the California wildflowers," blooms atop swaying stems taller than a man.

Midway down the final stretch is the mouth of Lost Woman Canyon, a tributary draining into Silverado Canyon from the south. When the wind whistles down this canyon, so the old-timers say, it evokes the plaintive sounds of a woman calling for help. Treading softly down the road, mildly hallucinating after many long miles, you may hear her.

Bent Coulter pine, Upper Silverado Canyon

TRIP 7 Harding Road to Laurel Spring

Distance	10.0 miles round trip, Out-and-back
Hiking Time	5½ hours (round trip)
Elevation Gain/Loss	2300'/2300'
Difficulty	Moderately strenuous
Trail Use	Dogs allowed, suitable for mountain biking
Best Times	October through May
Agency	CNF/TD
Optional Maps	USGS 7.5-min *Santiago Peak;* Cleveland National Forest recreation map
Notes	Marked trails/obvious routes, easy terrain

DIRECTIONS Exit from either eastern toll road (Highway 241 or 261) at Santiago Canyon Road. Drive 9 miles east and south to Modjeska Canyon Road, on the left. Proceed 2 miles to Tucker Wildlife Sanctuary and the start of the Harding Truck Trail, just short of the end of the road.

Tucked into an upper tributary of Santiago Canyon, Laurel Spring is a lofty mini-retreat just 3 air-miles from the expanding edge of Orange County's outer suburbs. While the surface flow at the spring merely fills a concrete watering trough, the abundant groundwater nourishes a thriving thicket of California bay (bay laurel) trees. Under the cathedral-like canopy of these trees, the cool, pungent odor of bay leaves wafts on the breeze like incense.

The long walk up to the spring on Harding Road is relieved—in the cooler, wetter months, at least—by the pleasure of the aromatic and sometimes colorful sage-scrub and chaparral vegetation. In spring, blue-flowering ceanothus and matilija poppies put on a great show. Harding Road (formerly called Harding Truck Trail) is passable for fire trucks, but normally closed to motorized traffic, with gates at both bottom (Modjeska Canyon) and top (Main Divide Road).

Early risers will appreciate this hike, especially in fall and early winter, when late sunrises make it convenient to hit the trail in time to enjoy a bit of stargazing before dawn's first light. Before the sun cleared the horizon one November morning, I ran into two other groups of hikers on the Harding Road with just that idea in mind.

Across from the Tucker sanctuary, the gated fire road signed 5S08 HARDING ROAD, begins curling up a hillside. Heading up this road on foot or by mountain bike, you soon pass into Cleveland National Forest. Ahead is a bold outcrop of conglomerate rock, consisting of sediments laid down in a marine environment roughly 80 million years ago. More of this erosion-resistant, cliff-forming layer will be seen on ridges to the north and south as you climb a little higher.

At a road fork in 0.4 mile, stay right; the left road goes down to Modjeska

Bush poppy, Main Divide Road

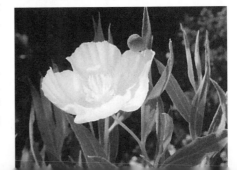

Reservoir and the mouth of Harding Canyon (see Trip 9). At 0.7 mile a ridgetop clearing next to a hairpin turn provides a view straight up the tree-choked bottom of Harding Canyon, a tributary of Santiago Canyon. The upper reaches of this seemingly impenetrable canyon were the scene of a short-lived mining boomlet shortly following the bigger boom in Silverado Canyon.

After 1.0 mile Harding Road descends about 100 feet (the only reversal in the steady ascent to Laurel Spring) in order to edge around a couple of steep ravines. Climbing again, you round the nose of a ridge and come upon (1.6 miles) the remnants of a wooden structure—known as the "goat shed" by local residents—over-looking the whole of Modjeska Canyon. To the east, a trench-like section of Santiago Canyon winds upward toward Old Saddleback.

The road continues generally east on or near the ridgeline dividing Harding and Santiago canyons. In early morning, the view behind is often that of cottony layers of fog or low clouds obscuring the coastal plain. The hum of traffic in the distant suburbs penetrates the murk.

At 4.9 miles a large landslide lies on the left. Just beyond, the road bends around the head of a ravine densely choked with bay laurel. On the right, look for the steep, narrow pathway that leads down about 50 vertical feet to Laurel Spring.

TRIP 8 Harding Road to Main Divide

Distance	19.0 miles round trip, Out-and-back
Hiking Time	9 hours (round trip)
Elevation Gain/Loss	3650'/3650'
Difficulty	Strenuous
Trail Use	Dogs allowed, suitable for mountain biking
Best Times	November through March
Agency	CNF/TD
Optional Maps	USGS 7.5-min *Santiago Peak;* Cleveland National Forest recreation map
Notes	Marked trails/obvious routes, easy terrain

DIRECTIONS Exit from either eastern toll road (Highway 241 or 261) at Santiago Canyon Road. Drive 9 miles east and south to Modjeska Canyon Road, on the left. Proceed 2 miles to Tucker Wildlife Sanctuary and the start of the Harding Road, just short of the end of Modjeska Canyon Road.

This challenging cool-weather trip is ideal for the exercise-minded, be they long-distance hikers, mountain runners, or mountain bicyclists. Since well over half this route stays on the north side of the ridgeline dividing Santiago and Harding canyons, the long shadows of late fall and winter provide plenty of welcome shade. There is also the distinct possibility, perhaps once every year or two, of skiing the upper part of Harding Road immediately following a cold, wet winter storm. (You would, of course, have to carry your cross-country skis perhaps 3 or more miles up the road to the first snow.)

Begin as in Trip 7. If you drop down from Harding Road to visit Laurel Spring (5.0 miles), you can get back to the road a little faster by following a 0.2-mile-long path that curls south and east from the spring and joins the road again.

At 6.0 miles Harding Road curls over to the north-facing side of the ridgeline and thereafter sticks to the slopes overlooking Harding Canyon. Dense chaparral—manzanita, scrub oak, mountain mahogany, and blue-flowering ceanothus (wild lilac)—mantles these slopes, but some Coulter pines and canyon live oaks rise above the shrubbery. In protected pockets both north and south of the road, small clusters of battered big-cone Douglas-firs have found a safe haven from the fires that periodically sweep through. In the larger, north-draining ravines, where moisture is retained in the soil, a smattering of small willows and sycamores can be seen.

Grotto Spring, at 8.6 miles, is usually completely dry. At 9.5 miles you reach Main Divide Road at a saddle overlooking the big drainage to the north—upper Silverado Canyon.

Options for further exploration include climbing Modjeska and Santiago peaks, which lie 1.3 miles and 2.4 miles away, respectively, via the shortest routes. Mountain cyclists can piece together a superb 27-mile ride by stringing together Harding and Maple Springs roads, then closing the loop via the paved Silverado Canyon, Santiago Canyon, and Modjeska Canyon roads.

TRIP 9 Harding Canyon

Distance	5.0 miles round trip, Out-and-back
Hiking Time	4 hours (round trip)
Elevation Gain/Loss	900'/900'
Difficulty	Moderately strenuous
Trail Use	Dogs allowed
Best Times	December through May
Agency	CNF/TD
Recommended Map	USGS 7.5-min *Santiago Peak*
Notes	Marked trails/obvious routes, difficult terrain

DIRECTIONS Exit from either eastern toll road (Highway 241 or 261) at Santiago Canyon Road. Drive 9 miles east and south to Modjeska Canyon Road, on the left. Proceed 2 miles to Tucker Wildlife Sanctuary and the start of the Harding Road, just short of the end of Modjeska Canyon Road.

In 1878 a pair of prospectors discovered some nodules containing lead and silver ore about 3 miles up Harding Canyon from the present-day Modjeska Reservoir. Soon miners swarmed so thickly throughout the canyon that, according to a newspaper account of the day, a man could hardly swing a pick without "perforating his neighbor."

The "Seven Pools hike" into the upper reaches Harding Canyon will simply amaze you—assuming you go in a year of normal rainfall or better, and before summer's heat and drought dries up the canyon's lively, crystalline, spring-fed stream. It's almost unbelievable that such a pristine place can exist just a few miles away from south Orange County's densely populated communities.

The canyon bottom features potentially ankle-busting terrain, so wear boots with ankle support. Also, poison oak grows in fair abundance along the banks of the stream, so consider applying a poison-ivy block to any exposed areas of your skin. You should budget four hours of moderate hiking and strenuous boulder-hopping for the round trip to the falls and pools—and more time than that if water levels are high.

You begin, as in Trips 7 and 8 above, by starting upward on Harding Road from Modjeska Canyon. After 0.4 mile, in a saddle along a ridge, Harding Road curves right to follow that ridge upward

Harding Canyon Creek in flood

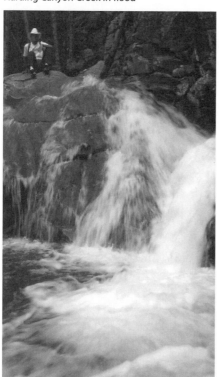

and a spur road descends left. Make the descent, and soon reach the broad flood plain of Harding Canyon just below its mouth. Turn right, go upstream alongside the tumbling (or trickling, as it may be) creek, and enter the canyon proper within about 0.2 mile.

Abandon the notion of trying to keep your feet dry if the water level is high. A sketchy use trail darts along either the right or the left bank, but you'll encounter plenty of ankle- to knee-deep stream crossings in between the trail segments. After periods of heavy rain, every ravine of any consequence along both sides of the canyon supports a lively brook rushing down to join the main stream. Live oaks, willows, and sycamores in the lower canyon are joined by aromatic bay laurels and straight-trunked white alder trees as you climb into the canyon's progressively narrower, higher reaches.

At about 1.5 miles into Harding Canyon, notice how the canyon walls morph from tan-and-beige-colored sedimentary rock to light-gray-colored granitic rock. At an abrupt bend to the left, where water sometimes sprays down a cliff-like ravine on the right, notice two mining prospects pocking the canyon wall on the left.

For a distance of several hundred yards ahead, cascades and deep aquamarine pools line the canyon bottom. The clarity of the water is remarkable, without a hint of turbidity or sudsing despite the churning flow. Enjoy the sights and sounds, take a dip if you like, then head back home.

TRIP 10 Santiago Trail

Distance	15.0 miles (to Old Camp and back), Out-and-back
Hiking Time	8 hours (round trip)
Elevation Gain/Loss	2650'/2650'
Difficulty	Moderately strenuous
Trail Use	Dogs allowed, suitable for mountain biking
Best Times	November through April
Agency	CNF/TD
Recommended Maps	USGS 7.5-min *El Toro, Santiago Peak;* or Cleveland National Forest recreation map
Notes	Marked trails/obvious routes, easy terrain

DIRECTIONS Exit from either eastern toll road (Highway 241 or 261) at Santiago Canyon Road. Drive 9 miles east and south to Modjeska Canyon Road, on the left. Proceed 0.9 mile to Modjeska Grade Road and turn right. Continue 0.7 mile to the top of the grade and the start of the Santiago Trail. (If you are coming from the south, this starting point is 0.5 mile north of Santiago Canyon Road.) Carefully observe the posted no-parking zones along Modjeska Grade Road when choosing a spot to park.

Yesteryear, Old Camp was a popular rendezvous point for hunting parties using the Joplin Trail between Rose Canyon and Old Saddleback. Now only remnants of the Joplin Trail remain, and Old Camp is simply a flat spot in Santiago Canyon shaded by massive live oaks, bay laurels, and bigleaf maples.

Old Camp retains its charm as a remote hideaway. It's well worth the day-long hike if the weather is cool. In late fall the maples really put on a show, and by winter or early spring the adjoining creek, screened by alders, bubbles with a delightfully pure flow of water.

Today Old Camp is reached by way of the Santiago Trail, a fire road closed to motor vehicles. Sticking close to the original Joplin route over part of its length, it runs for about 7 miles along the sunny ridgeline just south of Santiago Canyon, finally dropping abruptly into the canyon. The walk can be tedious at times, but there are diversions for the adventurous. At least four primitive pathways

descend into the depths of Santiago Canyon from points along the way, offering a taste of a moist, green, almost gloomy environment totally unlike the sunstruck one on the ridgeline.

Start by heading east on Santiago Trail, a fire road, and in a mile enter Cleveland National Forest. At 2.8 miles, you begin skirting the back side of the Vulture Crags. These broken outcrops of conglomerate rock served as a nesting site for California condors over a hundred years ago. On a little farther, you can look back and note, below the crags, layer upon layer of beige to brick-red marine sediments, all spectacularly tilted as a result of the rise of the Santa Ana Mountain crest to the east.

At 3.7 miles the Santiago Trail makes a bend at the 2400-foot contour, and a narrow, partially overgrown trail strikes off obliquely down the slope. This is the easiest and safest way to reach the canyon bottom short of Old Camp. In late fall a phantasmagoric pattern of bright maple leaves carpets the stream banks and limpid pools, and newly unfurled ferns adorn the lower slopes. Downstream, you can find evidence of mining (circa 1880) in the form of scattered bricks, cast-iron machine parts, prospect holes, and tailings mostly well hidden among the leaf litter and dense vegetation. Wear long pants if you poke around here: you'll probably run into some poison oak and scratchy chaparral. There's an active mining claim down in this part of the canyon, so be sure to respect the rights of the claim holder. Also remember that the old mining debris is considered historic and therefore legally protected against removal.

After 7.2 miles on the Santiago Trail, the road forks. A short spur road continues upward to follow a small powerline, while the Santiago Trail bears left and descends to Old Camp (7.5 miles). In addition to the variety of trees already mentioned, you'll find growths of wild blackberry, buckthorn ceanothus, redberry, coffee berry, and bracken fern in the area.

Further exploration in the area might proceed along the following lines: With the aid of the Santiago Peak topo map, it's possible to follow the upper part of the Joplin Trail as far as the low point (between Modjeska and Santiago peaks) in Old Saddleback. From Old Camp the trail threads through a shady tributary of Santiago Canyon, then gains a brush-covered slope, passing west of a 3893-foot knob. After winding amid some oaks, it angles up a steep slope thickly covered by chamise and buckthorn, a prickly variety of ceanothus. At about 1.3 miles from Old Camp, the trail descends a little, passes through a beautiful thicket of live oaks, bay laurels, and big-cone Douglas-fir, and returns to the bed of Santiago Canyon about 100 yards above Jamison Spring. Another 0.7 mile of ascent brings you to Main Divide Road atop the saddle.

The Joplin Trail is lightly maintained and therefore may be difficult to follow. Some hardy mountain bikers have discovered the trail, and that in itself has contributed to keeping it minimally clear of encroaching brush.

Mining debris, Santiago Canyon

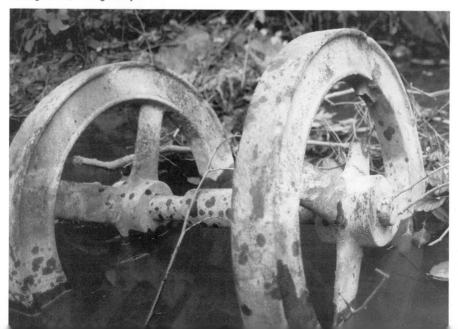

TRIP 11 Holy Jim Falls

Distance	2.8 miles round trip, Out-and-back
Hiking Time	1½ hours (round trip)
Elevation Gain/Loss	650'/650'
Difficulty	Moderate
Trail Use	Dogs allowed, good for kids
Best Times	November through June
Agency	CNF/TD
Optional Map	USGS 7.5-min *Santiago Peak*
Notes	Marked trails/obvious routes, easy terrain

DIRECTIONS From Trabuco Canyon Road, at the easternmost end of O'Neill Regional Park in Rancho Santa Margarita, turn east on the rough, unpaved Trabuco Creek Road. Proceed 4.7 miles to the Holy Jim Trailhead, on the left.

Sometimes the intimacy of a tiny, hidden waterfall is more aesthetically rewarding than the thunder of a famous one. Such is the case with Holy Jim Falls. Tucked into a short, steep canyon draining the southeast flank of Santiago Peak, the falls are seemingly remote but relatively easily reached on foot. The last stretch of trail leading to the falls may be a little overgrown with poison oak, so wear long pants and a long-sleeved shirt.

From the Holy Jim Trailhead, proceed up the road heading north into Holy Jim Canyon, passing more cabins beneath the sheltering trees. A century ago this canyon was home to settlers who eked out a living by raising bees. One beekeeper, James T. Smith, became so famous for his cursing habit that he was popularly named "Cussin' Jim." Other nicknames bestowed on him included "Lyin' Smith," "Greasy Jim," and "Salvation Smith." Dignified government cartographers invented a new one, "Holy Jim."

After 0.5 mile you come to a sturdy steel gate. Beyond, a narrow trail continues upstream, crossing the creek seven times in 0.7 mile. Typical moisture-loving

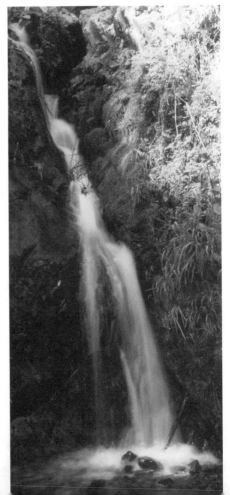

Holy Jim Falls

native trees, ferns, and chaparral shrubs line the canyon, but you'll also see naturalized fig trees and a purple-flowered ground cover called vinca (or periwinkle), the latter two introduced by the early settlers. Just after the last stream crossing, the trail switches back sharply to the left and begins ascending the west slope of the canyon. Leave the main trail at this point and continue straight up the bottom of the canyon on an even narrower trail. After about 400 yards you'll come to the shallow pool and grotto at the base of the falls. Above it the water cascades perhaps 18 feet over a broken cliff.

TRIP 12 Santiago Peak via Holy Jim Trail

Distance	15.0 miles round trip, Out-and-back
Hiking Time	9 hours (round trip)
Elevation Gain/Loss	3950'/3950'
Difficulty	Strenuous
Trail Use	Dogs allowed
Best Times	November through April
Agency	CNF/TD
Recommended Map	USGS 7.5-min *Santiago Peak*
Notes	Marked trails/obvious routes, easy terrain

DIRECTIONS From Trabuco Canyon Road, at the easternmost end of O'Neill Regional Park in Rancho Santa Margarita, turn east on the rough, unpaved Trabuco Creek Road. Proceed 4.7 miles to the Holy Jim Trailhead, on the left.

To the Indians, it was Kalawpa ("a wooded place"), the lofty resting place of the deity Chiningchinish. Early settlers and surveyors named it variously Mount Downey, Trabuco Peak, Temescal Mountain, and Santiago Peak. Finally, mapmakers decided on the name that eventually stuck: Santiago. Today's 'dozer-scraped summit overrun with telecommunications antennae hardly pays just homage to the peak's historic and scenic values. Witness, for example, this record of its first documented ascent in 1853, by a group of lawmen pursuing horse thieves up Coldwater Canyon:

After an infinite amount of scrambling, danger and hard labor, we stood on the very summit of the Temescal mountain, now by some called Santiago…where we beheld with pleasure a sublime view, more than worth the journey and ascent…

In 1861, while making a geologic survey of the Santa Anas, William Brewer and Josiah Whitney reached the same summit on their second try, using the ridge north of Coldwater Canyon. Their impressions echoed the sentiments of the earlier climbers: "The view more than repaid us for all we had endured."

The view so enthusiastically described by these early climbers is equally spectacular today—given, perhaps, a clearer-than-average winter day. Under good conditions, you can trace the coastline from Point Loma to Point Dume, spot both Santa Catalina Island and San

Clemente Island, and scratch your head trying to identify the plethora of mountain ranges and lesser promontories filling the landscape inland.

Clockwise around the compass from northwest to southeast the major ranges on the horizon are the Santa Monica, San Gabriel, San Bernardino, Little San Bernardino, San Jacinto, Santa Rosa, Palomar, and Cuyamaca mountains. To the south you might see several of the lower ranges along the Mexican border and perhaps glimpse the flat-topped summit of Table Mountain, a few miles inland from the Baja California coast. In the west and northwest, smog permitting, the flat urban tapestry spreads outward, spiked by the glass skyscrapers of downtown Los Angeles.

Don't underestimate the time required to bag Santiago Peak by way of the Holy Jim Trail. In winter, you'll need an early start to ensure a daylight return. With summit temperatures roughly 20 degrees cooler than below, you should pack along some extra clothing. Plenty of water is a good idea too: Bear Spring, on the way to the summit, should not be considered a potable source.

Begin this hike as in Trip 11 above, but continue following the main trail as it switchbacks up the chaparral-covered west wall of Holy Jim Canyon. Well traveled but minimally cleared of encroaching vegetation, the trail offers intimate glimpses of the immediate surroundings flashing by at eyeball level. Unlike walking on wide fire roads, there is a sense of motion and accomplishment as you ascend this trail.

Soon a few antenna structures atop Santiago Peak come into view, tantalizingly close, but about 3000 feet higher. At 2.7 miles, the trail crosses the bed of Holy Jim Canyon at elevation 3480 feet, well above the falls. You may be tempted at this point to follow the line of scattered trees that struggle up toward the head of the canyon, or try another short cut to the summit by way of the scree-covered slopes left or right; however, loose rock and thickets of thorny ceanothus would surely cost you more time, effort, and grief than you ever imagined.

So continue ahead on the trail, where soon you make a delicate traverse over an old landslide. After another mile on sunny, south-facing slopes, you contour around a ridge and suddenly enter a dark and shady recess filled with oaks, sycamores, bigleaf maples and big-cone Douglas-firs. By 4.5 miles, you come to Main Divide Road, opposite Bear Spring. Three more miles of steady climbing in sun and in shade along the Main Divide Road bring you to Santiago's summit.

You must walk around the antenna farm on the summit to take in the complete panorama. Modjeska Peak, one mile northwest and about 200 feet lower, isn't high enough to block the view of any far-horizon features. Modjeska and Santiago together make up the feature called "Old Saddleback" that appears exactly that shape when viewed from much of urban Orange County.

The fine-grained rock covering both summits of Old Saddleback is the prototype of the "Santiago Peak Volcanics" exposed on many of the coastal mountain ranges extending south through San Diego County into Baja California. These metamorphosed volcanic-rock formations were originally part of a chain of volcanic islands that collided with our continent some 80 million years ago.

TRIP 13 Indian Truck Trail

Distance	14.0 miles (to Main Divide and back), Out-and-back
Hiking Time	6½ hours (round trip)
Elevation Gain/Loss	2600'/2600'
Difficulty	Moderately strenuous
Best Times	November through April
Agency	CNF/TD
Optional Maps	USGS 7.5-min *Alberhill, Santiago Peak;* Cleveland National Forest recreation map
Notes	Marked trails/obvious routes, easy terrain

DIRECTIONS Leave Interstate 15 at the Indian Truck Trail exit south of Corona in Riverside County. Proceed 0.1 mile west, and turn right on Campbell Ranch Road. After 0.4 mile, turn left on Mayhew Canyon Road. Follow Mayhew Canyon Road 0.4 mile west, and follow the signs to the Indian Truck Trail access into Cleveland National Forest. (Note: these directions will likely change due to ongoing housing construction throughout the area.)

The most pleasant, if not shortest, way to hike to the Main Divide Road from the east is by way of Indian Truck Trail ("Indian Road" on some maps). Open intermittently to motor-vehicle traffic, it features easy grades throughout, considerable shade during the fall and winter months, and nice views because of its predominately ridgetop alignment. Hikers and mountain bikers have it all to themselves whenever the vehicle gate down at the bottom end is closed and locked.

On foot (or bike) now, you ascend gradually for about 0.4 mile and come to a road fork. A private road into a Korean church camp bears left; you stay right on the Indian Truck Trail. A vehicle gate, which may or may not be locked shut for vehicles, lies just ahead.

Upper Indian Truck Trail

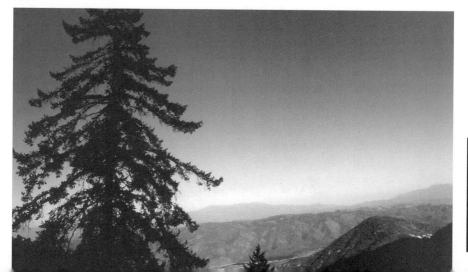

Your ascent quickens as Indian Truck Trail curls up the divide between Indian and Mayhew canyons. After about 3 miles in the sun, Indian Truck Trail makes a decided switch to the cool, north side of the ridge. Ferns grow in profusion along the shady road cuts, and the spreading limbs of live oaks and big-cone Douglas-firs frame a beautiful view of the Temescal Valley and the San Bernardino Mountains.

After about 5 miles, Indian Truck Trail traverses somewhat drier slopes, mantled with dense growths of manzanita and ceanothus and dotted with Coulter pines.

In the final two switchback legs, the road climbs to a saddle, joining (at 6.6 miles) Main Divide Road. Here you can look southwest toward the hills of southern Orange County and the coastline. On clear winter afternoons the glimmer of sunlight on the ocean's surface is breathtaking.

Indian Truck Trail, the Holy Jim Trail (Trip 12), and a short piece of Main Divide Road together make up an excellent transmountain hiking route. Total distance is 13 miles between the foot of Indian Truck Trail on the east side and the Holy Jim Trailhead on the west side.

TRIP 14 Trabuco Canyon

Distance	3.6 miles round trip, Out-and-back
Hiking Time	1½ hours (round trip)
Elevation Gain/Loss	850'/850'
Difficulty	Moderate
Trail Use	Dogs allowed, suitable for mountain biking, good for kids
Best Times	October through June
Agency	CNF/TD
Optional Maps	USGS 7.5-min *Santiago Peak, Alberhill*
Notes	Marked trails/obvious routes, easy terrain

DIRECTIONS From Trabuco Canyon Road, at the easternmost end of O'Neill Regional Park in Rancho Santa Margarita, turn east on the rough, unpaved Trabuco Creek Road. Proceed 5.7 miles to the end of the road.

Starting from the east terminus of Trabuco Creek Road, an old truck road turned narrow footpath meanders up to some of the most idyllic spots in the Santa Anas. Upper Trabuco Canyon is home to Orange County's biggest alder grove; to fine specimens of live oak, bay laurel, and maple; to a tiny community of madrones; and to a wide variety of spectacular spring wildflowers. Historically, the canyon is significant for its mining

activity, and as the site of the killing of California's last wild grizzly bear in 1908.

From there the trail passes under some large oaks, runs along the creekbed for a stretch, and then decidedly sticks to the sunny slope north of the creek. This slope is botanically best in late March and April, sporting colorful displays of bush lupine, matilija poppy, paintbrush, wild sweet pea, red and sticky monkeyflowers, prickly phlox, Mariposa lily, wild hyacinth, penstemon, and other spring flowers.

After 1.0 mile the trail passes close to an old adit, one of several reminders of gold-and-silver-mining activity, which persisted until about 1925. Some scraggly big-cone Douglas-fir trees can be seen on a darkly vegetated slope to the south, part of a small, privately owned inholding in the National Forest which includes Yaeger Mesa. Early miner Jake Yaeger built his cabin in the shade of a spreading maple down near the creek.

At 1.8 miles you come to the signed junction of the Horsethief Trail, half-concealed in thickets of brush and poison oak. Down below, the alder-shaded creekbed is a fine place to picnic or rest before heading back along the same trail. Read on for a description of an extended loop hike circling the head of Trabuco Canyon.

TRIP 15 West Horsethief-Trabuco Canyon Loop

Distance	10.0 miles, Loop
Hiking Time	6 hours
Elevation Gain/Loss	2700'/2700'
Difficulty	Moderately strenuous
Trail Use	Dogs allowed, suitable for mountain biking
Best Times	November through April
Agency	CNF/TD
Recommended Maps	USGS 7.5-min *Santiago Peak, Alberhill*
Notes	Marked trails/obvious routes, moderate terrain

DIRECTIONS From Trabuco Canyon Road, at the easternmost end of O'Neill Regional Park in Rancho Santa Margarita, turn east on the rough, unpaved Trabuco Creek Road. Proceed 5.7 miles to the end of the road.

The combination of wide-open views atop the Main Divide, and passages through pockets of dense chaparral and timber in the uppermost reaches of Trabuco Canyon make this one of the more varied and interesting hikes in this book.

You begin, as in Trip 14, with a steady climb 1.8 miles up Trabuco Canyon to a junction, with the West Horsethief Trail branching left. Take it. Earlier, you probably spotted switchbacks carving up the treeless slope that now lies east of you. These replaced the original straight-up-the-ridge route used by Indians in prehistoric times and by horse thieves in the Spanish days. Traffic by hikers and mountain bikers in recent years has helped keep today's trail clear of encroaching vegetation. Nonetheless, some sections are very rough and rocky. After following a canyon bottom for a short while, the West Horsethief Trail begins climbing in earnest, zigzagging through dense chaparral. During the coolness of the morning, diligent effort will get you to the top of this tedious stretch fast enough; later in the day this could be a hot, energy-sapping climb.

After 1100 feet of elevation gain the trail straightens, begins to level out along a ridge, and enters a vegetation zone dominated by manzanita and blue-flowering ceanothus. Cool "mountain" air washes over you, perhaps bearing the scent of the pines that lie ahead. Nearly coincident with the change of vegetation is a change in the rocks and soils underfoot. As you climb higher, light-colored granitic boulders and soil replace the dark-brown, crumbly metasedimentary rocks seen earlier. Although the younger granitic rock doesn't crop out below, you may remember having seen granitic boulders down in the bed of Trabuco Canyon. These resistant blocks, originally weathered out of the granitic mass above, were swept downhill during flash floods.

At 3.3 miles from the Trabuco Canyon roadhead, the Horsethief Trail joins Main Divide Road in a sparse grove of Coulter pines. Turn right and follow the road east, then south, for an easy, meandering, viewful 2.5 miles. On the left you will soon pass the East Horsethief Trail, currently "landlocked" by private property far below. During prehistoric times, the entire Horsethief Trail route was an important trans-mountain route from the coast to the inland valleys.

At 5.8 miles, amid a patch of Coulter pines and incense-cedars, you come to Los Pinos Saddle. At the northwest corner of a large, cleared area in the saddle itself, find the old roadbed (Trabuco Canyon Trail) angling downward along the shady slopes of Trabuco Canyon's main fork. Thick stands of live oak and big-cone Douglas-fir keep this part of the trail dark and gloomy during the fall and winter months, and delightfully cool at other times. Flowering currant and ceanothus shrubs at the trailside brighten things up in the spring.

One mile below the saddle, the trail veers left, crosses a divide, and begins descending along a tributary of Trabuco Canyon. You walk by thickets of California bay (bay laurel), which exude an enigmatically pleasant/pungent scent. After crossing the tributary ravine twice, the trail clings to a dry and sunny south-facing slope. Down below, in an almost inaccessible section of the ravine, you may hear water trickling and tumbling over boulders half-hidden under tangles of underbrush and trees. Before long, you arrive back at the junction of the Horsethief Trail in shady Trabuco Canyon, and continue down to the trailhead.

Inside Trabuco Canyon

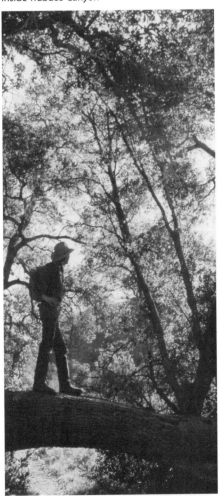

Chapter 13
Santa Ana Mountains—
Ortega Corridor

From San Juan Capistrano to Lake Elsinore, Highway 74—Ortega Highway—stretches like a snake over the midsection of the Santa Ana Mountains. Leisurely rising from the west through San Juan Canyon to the oak-dotted crest, then descending the east escarpment via sharp curves, the road gives casual drivers their only glimpse of the interior Santa Anas.

The highway commemorates Jose Francisco Ortega, sergeant and scout in the Portola party, which in 1769 passed through Orange County's coastal hills while heading up the California coast. The present roadway, completed in 1933, followed a turn-of-the-century wagon track, which in turn evolved from the route of a centuries-old Juaneno Indian Trail. The highway's rustic character remains, much to the delight of the unhurried sightseer but not the growing numbers of frustrated commuters who race along it daily to and from employment centers in southern Orange County.

The Forest Service recognizes Ortega Highway as an important recreational corridor. Campground facilities have

View from Ortega Summit

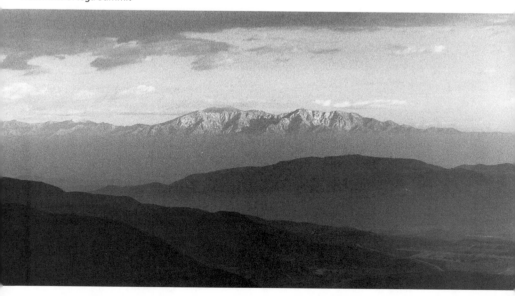

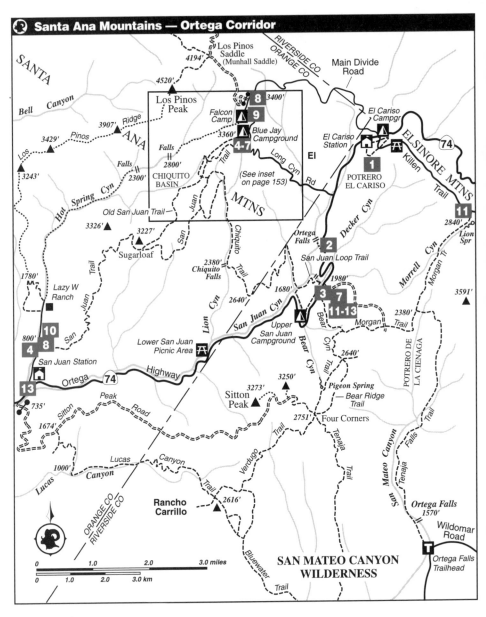

been constructed and several trailheads have been developed. But few roads penetrate the backcountry areas, and foot trails are the usual way of getting around.

Dayhiking (along with mountain biking and horseback riding) and car camping are popular in the Ortega Corridor. Overnight backpacking is allowed south of the highway, but only within San Mateo Canyon Wilderness (see Chapter 14 for complete coverage of this area).

Roadside camping facilities are found at Caspers Wilderness Park (Chapter 10), and in several areas within the national forest. The national-forest facilities include the always-open El Cariso Campground

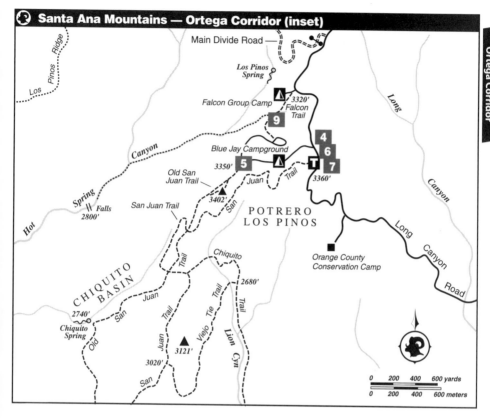

and the seasonally open Upper San Juan Campground. Both lie along Ortega Highway and therefore can get considerable traffic noise. Delightful and secluded Blue Jay Campground rests high in the remote Potrero Los Pinos area, north of Ortega Highway. Blue Jay Campground and its neighbor, Falcon Group Camp (for large groups with reservations), are open seasonally, from May until November.

The drive up Ortega Highway is an enjoyable prelude to a day's hiking activities. Starting from the San Juan Capistrano side, the highway runs through outlying suburban development, rolling hills still used for grazing, and the rugged foothills of Caspers Wilderness Park. Past Caspers you come to San Juan Fire Station and the national-forest boundary. On ahead Ortega Highway winds along the precipitous south wall of San Juan Canyon, passing Lower San Juan Picnic Area and Upper San Juan Campground. A major trailhead is located next to the Ortega Country Cottage (aka, Candy Store), 0.7 mile past Upper San Juan Campground. From here, trails lead north into the Potrero Los Pinos area and south into San Mateo Canyon Wilderness.

After another 2.5 miles, Ortega Highway levels out in a pleasant oak woodland (Potrero El Cariso). Long Canyon Road, intersecting on the left (west), climbs higher to another oak-dotted area—Potrero Los Pinos—and Blue Jay Campground. A little over a mile past Long Canyon Road, Ortega Highway passes the El Cariso ranger station and visitor center (open daily; maps and information available) and El Cariso Campground.

Just east of that, Main Divide Road (renamed the Killen Trail on the south side of the highway) crosses Ortega Highway, providing access to areas along the Main Divide of the Santa Ana Mountains to the north, and to the Elsinore Mountains to the south. A little farther on, Ortega Highway begins its abrupt descent to Lake Elsinore. Wending your way through the community of Lake Elsinore, you can pick up Interstate 15, which will take you back to Orange County if you use I-15 north and take the Riverside Freeway (Highway 91) west at Corona.

TRIP 1 El Cariso Nature Trail

Distance	1.3 miles, Loop
Hiking Time	1 hour
Elevation Gain/Loss	150'/150'
Difficulty	Easy
Trail Use	Dogs allowed, good for kids
Best Times	All year
Agency	CNF/TD
Optional Map	USGS 7.5-min *Alberhill*
Notes	Marked trails/obvious routes, easy terrain

DIRECTIONS Park at the El Cariso Fire Station and Visitor Center, on the south side of Ortega Highway, 23 miles east of Interstate 5 at San Juan Capistrano and about 6 miles west of Lake Elsinore.

If you're not very familiar with the natural history of the Santa Ana Mountains, stop first at El Cariso visitor center along Ortega Highway. Inside the small visitor center here you'll find some small but instructive exhibits on the local flora, fauna, and geology. To learn even more pick up the El Cariso Nature Trail self-guiding leaflet, then walk the trail itself, which begins just behind the visitor building. Anyone making a brief stop at the visitor station need not display a National Forest Adventure Pass, but anyone using the trail is supposed to.

The opportunity to become familiar with common varieties of native shrubs is the real value of taking this short walk. You'll see examples of chamise, buckwheat, manzanita, scrub oak, sugar bush, and three types of sage. In spring, monkeyflower, blue-eyed grass, nightshade, and other vivid-hued annual flowers compete for attention, while the blooms of wild peony nod circumspectly close to the ground. Amid the tangled branches of the shrubs look for the spiny, green fruits of the wild cucumber.

At the start of the trail, miner's lettuce (in winter and spring) coats the shady ground almost like a manicured lawn. There's a brief passage under some oaks, then the trail begins winding moderately upward on a chaparral- and sage-covered slope. The view to the west is of rolling country dotted with small houses on large lots (the area around El Cariso is a patchwork of national-forest and private lands).

Soon the trail levels out and turns east to circle a hilltop, passing an old mine shaft. Then it descends slightly to cross the Killen Trail (a paved road). Continue diagonally across the road and pick up the remainder of the trail, harder to follow now. After meandering through a grove of "Penny Pines"—Coulter pines, plus some oak and cypress trees—you arrive back at the starting point.

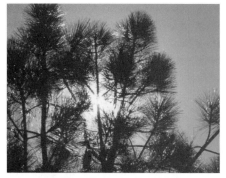

Coulter pines, El Cariso Nature Trail

TRIP 2 Ortega Falls

Distance	0.5 mile round trip, Out-and-back
Hiking Time	1 hour (round trip)
Elevation Gain/Loss	200'/200'
Difficulty	Moderate
Trail Use	Dogs allowed, good for kids
Best Times	December through May
Agency	CNF/TD
Optional Map	USGS 7.5-min *Alberhill*
Notes	Marked trails/obvious routes, moderate terrain

DIRECTIONS Park at a wide turnout on the west side of Ortega Highway (mile 4.4 in Riverside County), 21 miles east of Interstate 5 at San Juan Capistrano and about 8 miles west of Lake Elsinore.

Often dry or merely trickling, Ortega Falls can come to life for days or for weeks following any significant winter storm. During the unusually wet years of 1998 and 2005, when the region received double or more the normal precipitation, these falls managed to put on an impressive show until May or June.

The unmarked trailhead is a wide turnout on the west side of Ortega Highway, 2.1 mile south of the El Cariso visitor center, and 1.5 mile north of the Candy Store or San Juan Loop Trail trailhead. According to the roadside highway markers stenciled "Riv" for Riverside County, the turnout is located at mile 4.4. Yes, you'll need to display a National Forest Adventure Pass on your parked car.

The hike to the falls is almost trivially short, but not quite a piece of cake, particularly for small kids. Follow the unmarked use trail descending through brush and boulders and down a steep draw to the boulder-choked streambed of Long Canyon, which is an upper tributary of San Juan canyon and creek. You turn upstream and make your way, preferably on the right bank, over sand, matted-down vegetation, and rocks. When the water is high, it may be easier to wade in a couple of spots rather than to boulder hop. Beyond a series of smaller cascades, you'll arrive at the foot of the main waterfall, which drops about 35 feet over a blocky granitic outcrop. Rock climbers sometimes practice on the sheer rock faces here, and it's obvious and unfortunate that spray-paint vandals also visit from time to time.

Ortega Falls

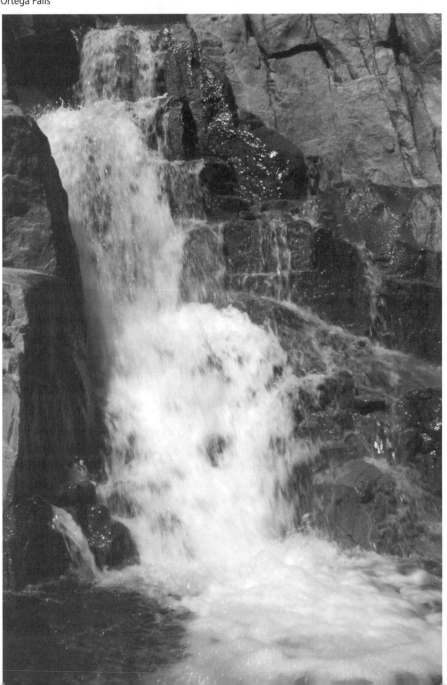

TRIP 3 San Juan Loop Trail

Distance	2.1 miles, Loop
Hiking Time	1 hour
Elevation Gain/Loss	350'/350'
Difficulty	Easy
Trail Use	Dogs allowed, suitable for mountain biking, good for kids
Best Times	October through June
Agency	CNF/TD
Optional Map	USGS 7.5-min *Sitton Peak*
Notes	Marked trails/obvious routes, easy terrain

DIRECTIONS Park opposite the "Candy Store" on Ortega Highway, 21 miles east of Interstate 5 at San Juan Capistrano and about 10 miles west of Lake Elsinore.

If you've no more time to spare than an hour while cruising the Ortega Highway, at least stop and try the San Juan Loop Trail (not to be confused with the much longer San Juan Trail, Trip 4). Sights include a small waterfall along San Juan Creek, excellent wildflower displays in the spring, and some of the finest oak woodland in the Santa Anas.

Park in the large trailhead parking lot (Adventure Pass needed) directly across from the Ortega Country Cottage—or as its been referred to for decades—the "Candy Store." From here pick up the well-worn path leading north, slightly uphill, along the slope overlooking the highway. After curving left and dropping a little, the trail threads the side of a narrow gorge resounding—in the wet season at least—with falling water. A spur trail leads down toward the lip of the falls; from there you can hop over to a reflecting pool and maybe settle into the polished granite for a moment's quiet meditation. A gnarled juniper clings sentinel-like to a bouldered slope overlooking the pool, far from its usual habitat on desert slopes 50 or more miles north and east.

San Juan Loop Trail

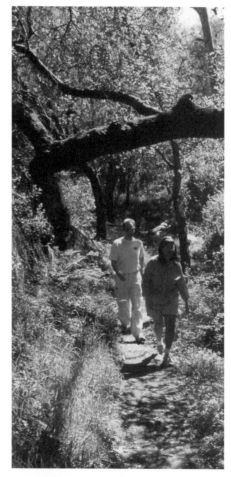

From the falls area, you descend on easy switchbacks through the chaparral and reach, after more than a half mile, an oak-dotted flat along San Juan Creek. Soon the Chiquito Trail branches north to cross the creek. The loop trail bears left (south) to follow Bear Canyon beside Ortega Highway. For a delightful few minutes as you walk here, the sky's brilliance is muted by the arching limbs of centuries-old live oaks, and the soft ground on the trailside is aglow with the seasonal greens, browns, and reds of ferns, poison-oak leaves, and wild grasses.

After touching briefly upon the outermost campsites of Upper San Juan Campground, the trail veers sharply left to gain an open slope. It may be easy to lose the trail here because of various side paths worn in by campers and confused hikers. Continue for another 0.5 mile across this sun-struck slope more or less parallel to Ortega Highway, and arrive back at the parking lot.

The San Juan Loop Trail has become quite rough and rocky in spots from decades of use. Part of or all of the trail, however, is scheduled to be upgraded to wheelchair-accessible status in the near future.

TRIP 4 San Juan Trail

Distance	11 miles, Point-to-point
Hiking Time	5 hours
Elevation Gain/Loss	550'/3100'
Difficulty	Moderately strenuous
Trail Use	Dogs allowed, suitable for mountain biking
Best Times	November through May
Agency	CNF/TD
Optional Maps	Cleveland National Forest recreation map;
	USGS 7.5-min *Alberhill, Sitton Peak, Canada Gobernadora*
Notes	Marked trails/obvious routes, easy terrain

DIRECTIONS EAST END: At a point on Ortega Highway 21.7 miles east of Interstate 5 at San Juan Capistrano (and about 7 miles west of Lake Elsinore), turn west on Long Canyon Road. Proceed 2.5 miles to upper end of the San Juan Trail, which lies just short of the entrance to Blue Jay Campground. WEST END: At a point on Ortega Highway 12.5 miles east of Interstate 5 at San Juan Capistrano, turn north on Hot Springs Canyon Road. Continue 0.8 mile north to the San Juan Trailhead.

With gentle grades most of the way, the San Juan Trail is tailor-made for a leisurely saunter from the Main Divide of the Santa Anas to the lower foothills. In recent years the trail has received a lot more use among mountain bikers. Since the trail runs largely along dry ridgelines exposed to the sun, hot days should be scrupulously avoided—unless you're willing to carry a lot of water and sweat copiously. Clear winter days bring out the best in the scenery. On some occasions the view takes in much of the southern Orange County coastline and Santa Catalina and San Clemente islands. Due to an elevation change of about 2500 feet, most of the spring wildflowers common to the chaparral and sage-scrub plant communities can be seen somewhere and sometime along this trail.

In this description I'll route you along the newer version of the San Juan Trail, originally an Indian trail but now built to modern standards with switchbacks

Alder thicket in Hot Spring Canyon

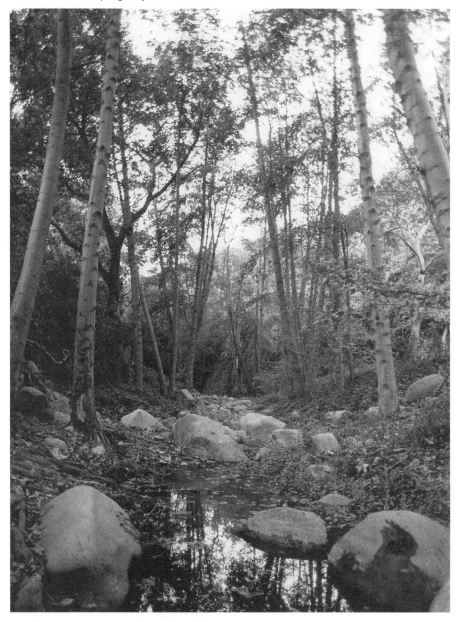

where needed. Shortcuts using older and more direct sections of the trail (shown on the Ortega Corridor inset map, page 153) may be taken if you want to save a little time.

Begin at the roadside trailhead and parking area 100 yards south of the entrance to Blue Jay Campground. From here the "new" San Juan Trail winds west and south around the heads of two shady canyons, just below the level of the campground. After about one mile, the trail starts descending along a sunny, sage-carpeted slope. At 1.3 miles the new trail, the one you're on, crosses the old trail, a steep, rocky roadbed, and plunges into the deep shade of a ravine. For a time, live oaks keep the sun's rays at bay.

After rounding a single switchback and descending further, you reach, in a sunny, sage-dotted clearing at 1.7 miles, a second crossing of the old trail, which from here leads to Chiquito Basin and then back up to join the new trail again just below Sugarloaf Peak. Keep straight and come to a junction, 1.8 miles, with the Chiquito Trail. Stay right here.

Continue south along the base of a hillside, through some tall and dense chaparral. Climbing slightly into a more sparsely vegetated zone, you arrive, 2.4 miles (3020′), at another junction, where the San Juan Trail bends right to cross the top of a gentle divide, and the Viejo Tie Trail, on the left, goes along the hillside.

Stay on the San Juan Trail, which now bears south-southwest through more chaparral. Reaching some oaks in a ravine bottom (3.7 miles), the trail zigzags a couple of times through grass and poison oak and crosses an intermittent stream. Enjoy the shade: this is the last grove of trees until you come to the end of the trail in Hot Spring Canyon.

On the far side of the ravine, the trail swings south of a peaklet (2966′), and then climbs moderately toward a flat area (5.0 miles) just south of Sugarloaf, where the old trail, a rutted firebreak at this point, comes in from the right. A short but tough climb to Sugarloaf's summit can be made from here, over big granitic boulders and through brush.

After dropping down along the west slope of Sugarloaf, you come to a saddle overlooking Hot Spring Canyon to the north. In the distant north, you'll spot the flat-topped, antenna-crowded summit of Santiago Peak.

The gradual descent continues, largely on or near the spine of a ridge offering nice views of other ridges and canyons in every direction. Far below to the south, the gray blacktop of Ortega Highway resembles a giant snake propelling itself through the sycamores in San Juan Canyon.

The granite boulders and decomposed granite soil seen earlier along the trail are not here; the trail now is hewn into friable metasedimentary rock, the same kind of metamorphosed sea-floor sediment typically found in Silverado and Trabuco canyons to the north.

At around 8.5 miles, several switchbacks take you safely down a crumbling slope. East of these switchbacks, a sharply folded anticline can be seen in the rock strata. To the west, other switchbacks on an earlier version of the trail can be spotted. At 10.0 miles, with only a mile to go, you begin descending quickly. A final set of zigzags takes you down into Hot Spring Canyon, where the trail intersects the road coming up from San Juan Fire Station.

TRIP 5 Chiquito Basin

Distance	2.8 miles round trip, Out-and-back
Hiking Time	2 hours (round trip)
Elevation Gain/Loss	700'/700'
Difficulty	Moderate
Trail Use	Dogs allowed, good for kids
Best Times	All year
Agency	CNF/TD
Optional Map	USGS 7.5-min *Alberhill*
Notes	Marked trails/obvious routes, easy terrain

DIRECTIONS At a point on Ortega Highway 21.7 miles east of Interstate 5 at San Juan Capistrano (and about 7 miles west of Lake Elsinore), turn west on Long Canyon Road. Proceed 2.5 miles to Blue Jay Campground, on the left.

If you want to spot wildlife, the earlier you make the hike to Chiquito Basin, the better. One morning, in the soft wet ground along the way, I discovered fresh tracks of a deer and a mountain lion, both apparently moving along at a running gait. With an earlier start I might have witnessed a terrific chase. It might bear repeating that in this remote corner of Orange County, as well as in the parklands of the lower foothills, mountain lions are occasionally spotted and attacks on hikers and mountain bikers have occurred. To stay as safe as possible, travel in groups and don't let kids stray.

Bedrock morteros, Chiquito Basin

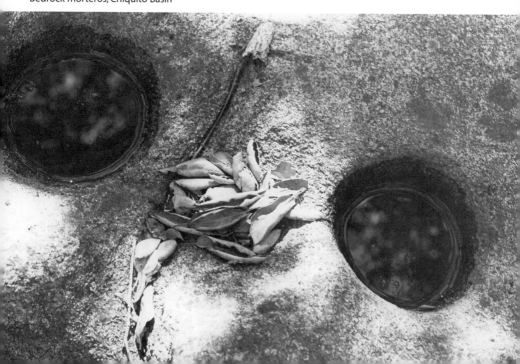

Start hiking from the west edge of Blue Jay Campground, 0.4 mile west of the entrance, and take the most direct route to Chiquito Basin—the old San Juan Trail. If the campground is closed (winter months), park outside the gate and pick up the new San Juan Trail skirting the campground (see Trip 4), or simply walk through the campground itself to reach the beginning of the old trail at the campground's west end. Either way, don't forget to display an Adventure Pass on your parked car.

The wide, rocky path of the old San Juan Trail leads southwest along the ridgeline past some walk-in campsites shaded by oaks and tall chaparral, and then pitches downhill. At 0.6 mile and again at 0.8 mile the new San Juan Trail, with its gentler but longer grade, crosses the old one. Keep straight to save time. Between these two crossings, white sage uniformly carpets the slopes on both sides of the old trail; in springtime its dull, grayish foliage is upstaged by Indian paintbrush, a plant thought to be parasitic on the roots of sage.

Continue downhill into the oak-rimmed meadow informally called Chiquito Basin. This is a great place for birdwatching, picnicking, or loafing. From the western corner of the meadow a faint trail leads to Chiquito Spring, named by early Cleveland Forest ranger Kenneth Munhall, who stopped there one warm afternoon in 1927 with his horse, Chiquito. The spring is bedecked with giant chain ferns and poison-oak vines, and buzzes with insects. On the poison-oak-infested slope north of the spring, you can find at least half a dozen morteros—Indian grinding holes worn into the granitic bedrock.

Return the same way, or if the spirit moves you, explore further. From the edge of Chiquito Basin, the old San Juan Trail veers south and climbs 300 vertical feet up a steep, oak-shaded slope to reach an open ridgetop offering a fine view of the basin and its surroundings. The old trail then turns southwest along this ridgeline and connects with the new San Juan Trail at the base of Sugarloaf peak. From here you might loop back to Blue Jay Campground by following the twists and turns of the new trail, if you have time.

TRIP 6 Viejo Tie Loop

Distance	5.5 miles, Loop
Hiking Time	3 hours
Elevation Gain/Loss	1000'/1000'
Difficulty	Moderate
Trail Use	Dogs allowed, suitable for mountain biking
Best Times	November through June
Agency	CNF/TD
Optional Map	USGS 7.5-min *Alberhill*
Notes	Marked trails/obvious routes, easy terrain

DIRECTIONS At a point on Ortega Highway 21.7 miles east of Interstate 5 at San Juan Capistrano (and about 7 miles west of Lake Elsinore), turn west on Long Canyon Road. Proceed 2.5 miles to upper end of the San Juan Trail, which lies just short of the entrance to Blue Jay Campground.

In Orange County the most dependable and most lavish displays of springtime flowering take place in the chaparral plant community. Beginning with the longer days and warmer soil temperatures of March, and ending with the onset of heat and drought in May or June, the higher mountains are alive with the color and fragrance of blooming plants large and small.

This hike takes you into stands of mature chaparral, dotted here and there with live oak trees. Aside from the common white-blooming ceanothus, you may discover at the trailside more than a dozen kinds of wildflowers. Typical finds are red monkeyflower, nightshade, prickly phlox, aster, golden yarrow, cow parsnip, wild pea, wild hyacinth, Indian pink, and Mariposa lily.

Begin as in Trip 4 above, taking the new San Juan Trail for 2.4 miles. Then bear left on the Viejo Tie Trail. After swinging left around the brow of a ridge, you descend northward through tall chaparral to reach the oak-shaded bed of Lion Canyon. On the far bank, after a couple of switchbacks, you come to the Chiquito Trail. Turn left, climb 300 vertical feet back to the San Juan Trail, crossing the creek bed again, and return the way you came.

TRIP 7 Chiquito Trail

Distance	9.2 miles, Point-to-point
Hiking Time	5 hours
Elevation Gain/Loss	900'/2300'
Difficulty	Moderately strenuous
Trail Use	Dogs allowed, suitable for mountain biking
Best Times	November through May
Agency	CNF/TD
Optional Maps	USGS 7.5-min *Alberhill, Sitton Peak*
Notes	Marked trails/obvious routes, easy terrain

DIRECTIONS NORTH END: At a point on Ortega Highway 21.7 miles east of Interstate 5 at San Juan Capistrano (and about 7 miles west of Lake Elsinore), turn west on Long Canyon Road. Proceed 2.5 miles to upper end of the San Juan Trail, which lies just short of the entrance to Blue Jay Campground. SOUTH END: The trip ends at the San Juan Loop Trail parking lot, opposite the "Candy Store" on Ortega Highway, 21 miles east of Interstate 5 at San Juan Capistrano and about 10 miles west of Lake Elsinore.

Like the San Juan Trail, the Chiquito Trail is best explored from end to end, downhill direction preferred. Along the way you'll enjoy cool passages through canyon bottoms, but also endure (if the weather is warm) a seemingly endless traverse across a sun-blasted ridge.

Completed in 1974, the Chiquito Trail is easy to follow, yet it's potentially an ankle-twister. In places sharp rocks have eroded out of the decomposed granite bed of the trail, so it's necessary to watch your step.

Begin at the upper terminus of the San Juan Trail (see Trip 3) and descend, using the easy switchbacks, to the Chiquito Trail junction, 1.8 miles. Turn left (east) and descend into Lion Canyon, 0.2 mile away. The canyon has water about half the year.

The next couple of miles down-canyon are delightful, with patchy shade provided by large oaks—the survivors of wildfires—and young sycamores. On the banks of the creek you'll find poison oak, wild blackberry, toyon, barberry, and ceanothus. Profuse displays of monkeyflower brighten the scene in April. The red monkeyflower and the sticky (yellow-flowered) monkeyflower may have hybridized here: the spectrum of monkeyflower colors includes orange, pink, and magenta, as well as the usual scarlet and light-yellow hues.

At 4.2 miles the trail makes an abrupt bend to the left and begins a long traverse across the ridge to the east. Just below this bend is Chiquito Falls, where the stream drops about 15 feet over an outcrop of granite. Impressive only after heavy rains, the site is a pleasant one anytime for a picnic.

Rising through scrubby chaparral and granitic boulders, the trail works around to a south-facing slope. The din of traffic from Ortega Highway less than one bee-line mile away is enough to convince you the end is near, but it's not. Instead, the trail curves northeast and crookedly descends for another 2 miles to an unnamed tributary of San Juan Canyon. To occupy yourself on the way down, look for hawks and golden eagles riding the thermals, and squirrels or lizards scurrying around at ground level.

Upon reaching the bottom of the unnamed canyon, the trail turns south to follow an intermittent watercourse, simi-lar to the creek in Lion Canyon. After another mile, you come to San Juan Canyon and the San Juan Loop Trail. Go either right or left around the loop to reach the large trailhead parking lot opposite the Candy Store.

TRIP 8 Los Pinos Ridge

Distance	10.5 miles, Point-to-point
Hiking Time	7 hours
Elevation Gain/Loss	2550'/5200'
Difficulty	Strenuous
Best Times	November through April
Agency	CNF/TD
Recommended Maps	USGS 7.5-min *Alberhill, Santiago Peak, Canada Gobernadora*
Notes	Navigation required, bushwhacking, moderate terrain

DIRECTIONS NORTH END: At a point on Ortega Highway 21.7 miles east of Interstate 5 at San Juan Capistrano (and about 7 miles west of Lake Elsinore), turn west on Long Canyon Road. Proceed 3.5 miles west and north to Main Divide Road (dirt truck trail) on the left. SOUTH END: At a point on Ortega Highway 12.5 miles east of Interstate 5 at San Juan Capistrano, turn north on Hot Springs Canyon Road. Continue 0.8 mile north to the San Juan Trailhead.

Although plotted as a trail on Forest Service and topographic maps, the Los Pinos ridge route has for decades received only irregular or no mainte-nance. Once a wide firebreak, it now serves as a throughway only for wildlife and a few adventurous humans. Clinging religiously to the undulating ridgeline, the route is tiring in its many uphills as well as its absurdly steep downhills. Prospective hikers should be ready to do battle with brush, and be equipped with tough trousers and sturdy shoes. Rat-tlesnakes may be a problem in warm weather; proceed slowly and cautiously through areas where you can't see the ground.

The greatest reward during the hike is the fine views west and south to the Pacific Ocean and the islands, east past Lake Elsinore to the highest summits of the Peninsular Ranges, and down into the V-shaped upper gorges of Hot Spring and Bell canyons.

The Los Pinos Trail is designated by the Forest Service as "landlocked," which means that there is no public access at its lower end. If you plan to hike this route all the way through, as I describe here, you'll need permission to pass through the Lazy W Ranch church camp (P.O. Box 579, San Juan Capistrano 92675; phone 949-728-0141; website www.lazywranch .org) at the lower end of the trail. Parking is limited and probably unavailable at the church camp itself.

From the north-end starting point, trudge up the steep road 1.7 miles to Los

Pinos Saddle (aka Munhall Saddle), where the Trabuco Canyon Trail joins Main Divide Road. Follow the wide firebreak going very steeply up the ridge to the southwest. The crumbly metasedimentary rock on the slope is a foretaste of what you will have to contend with in the miles ahead. Chamise, bush poppy, ceanothus, manzanita, and scattered Coulter pines keep a low profile along the ridge, allowing clear vistas in nearly every direction.

A mile from the saddle, you pass some fantastically weathered outcrops—part of a small exposure of the Santiago Peak Volcanics formation in this area. Nearby are surveyor's bench marks identifying Los Pinos Peak, fourth-highest named peak in the Santa Ana Mountains. (The three highest peaks—Santiago, Modjeska, and Trabuco—are on the Main Divide.) The true summit of the peak (elevation 4520+ feet) lies a little to the northeast of the bench marks.

Beyond Los Pinos Peak, the trail deteriorates. Over the next 3 miles, make sure you stay on the well-defined ridge between Hot Spring and Bell canyons. Scattered big-cone Douglas-firs struggle up the north-facing slopes, where the sun's drying effects are allayed. Coastal fog or haze sometimes fills the canyon bottoms. With the relief between ridgetop and canyon bottoms a somewhat sheer 1500 feet, you seem perched between two yawning abysses.

More and more chaparral and weedy plants choke the trail as you descend. As you grope through the brush just past Peak 3429, be very careful to stay on the correct ridgeline: here the route turns south to follow the ridge between Cold Spring Canyon and a tributary of Hot Spring Canyon.

As you descend into a secluded little bowl drained by Cold Spring Canyon, the trail condition may improve. This section has in the past been cleared and maintained by members of the church camp. Eventually, you'll come to a trail junction. Go either way: straight ahead takes you along the ridgeline and then straight down to the lower end of the church property; left takes you down multiple switchbacks to the upper end of the camp. Wend your way through the camp, past the entrance, and then down the road to the parking lot at the west terminus of the San Juan Trail.

TRIP 9 Upper Hot Spring Canyon

Distance	3.0 miles round trip, Out-and-back
Hiking Time	2 ½ hours (round trip)
Elevation Gain/Loss	450'/450'
Difficulty	Moderately strenuous
Trail Use	Dogs allowed
Best Times	December through May
Agency	CNF/TD
Recommended Map	USGS 7.5-min *Alberhill*
Notes	Navigation required, bushwhacking, moderate terrain

DIRECTIONS At a point on Ortega Highway 21.7 miles east of Interstate 5 at San Juan Capistrano (and about 7 miles west of Lake Elsinore), turn west on Long Canyon Road. Proceed 2.5 miles to Blue Jay Campground, on the left.

Silent, except for the gentle gurgle of water over stone, upper Hot Spring Canyon is an easy-to-reach retreat not far from the popular campgrounds in the Potrero Los Pinos area. Boulder-hopping and mild bushwhacking take you to an interesting area of small waterfalls and dark, limpid pools.

Start at either campground—Blue Jay or Falcon—and walk about halfway out the Falcon Trail, which connects the two. From there, drop down into a shallow gully to the west, using any one of several informal paths. Follow this gully downstream, dodging brush along the way. You'll soon join a bigger gully at the head of Hot Spring Canyon carrying water from Los Pinos Spring, which lies a short distance upstream. Memorize or mark this junction for the trip back.

A narrow, lightly beaten path goes down-canyon along grassy benches and across crumbly metasedimentary rock, crossing the creek several times. The canyon ahead trends consistently southwest, despite a few bends. You're following the Los Pinos Fault, an inactive fault running perpendicular to the Elsinore Fault and other faults responsible for the

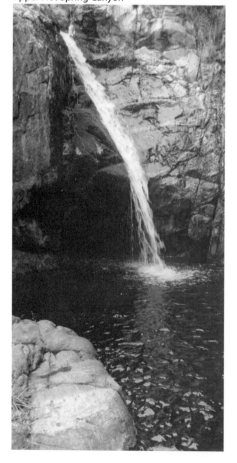

Falls in metamorphic rock, upper Hot Spring Canyon

recent (in a geological sense) uplift of the Santa Ana Mountains.

Just before you reach the junction of a major, wet canyon to the north (2950′), there's a small waterfall and a grotto with two shallow pools. On the rocks, ferns, mosses, and a type of succulent "live-for-ever" descriptively known as "lady fingers" add to the charm. A cluster of alders grows nearby; they are found in increasing numbers downstream, all the way to San Juan Canyon.

After another 0.4 mile, the canyon bottom makes a bend to the right and drops abruptly. All but experienced climbers should stop here and go no farther. Intrepid climbers may want to try (very cautiously) working their way over the loose metamorphic rock ahead to get a glimpse of a hidden 25-foot waterfall and a deep pool. Below this, the water shoots down a slot through polished granite. (Note: The rock in this area is very loose and unstable. Standard rock-climbing techniques are of little value.)

Further progress down-canyon toward the big falls (read on—Trip 10) is possible only by long and difficult traverses over the canyon walls to either side.

TRIP 10 Lower Hot Spring Canyon

Distance	9.0 miles (to falls and back), Out-and-back
Hiking Time	10 hours (round trip)
Elevation Gain/Loss	1600′/1600′
Difficulty	Strenuous
Best Times	December through March
Agency	CNF/TD
Recommended Maps	USGS 7.5-min *Canada Gobernadora, Santiago Peak, Alberhill*
Notes	Navigation required, bushwhacking, difficult terrain

DIRECTIONS   At a point on Ortega Highway 12.5 miles east of Interstate 5 at San Juan Capistrano, turn north on Hot Springs Canyon Road. Continue 0.8 mile north to the San Juan Trailhead.

This is a trip of superlatives—arguably the most beautiful canyon hike in the Santa Ana Mountains, and arduous to boot. The goal is a magnificent 140-foot waterfall, one of Southern California's highest. This is also a deceptively difficult hike—in fact, it's the most strenuous, and objectively the most hazardous, of all the trips in this book.

Being in excellent physical condition, having considerable experience in cross-country travel over rugged terrain, and possessing good judgment do not automatically guarantee that you'll be able to reach the falls and return without mishap. You must be cautious, patient, and determined too. Hazards include slippery rocks (some concealed by leaf litter), prickly vegetation, and forests of poison oak. Long pants, a long-sleeved shirt, and sturdy boots are musts.

Several factors determine the appropriate time of year to take this trip. Autumn leaves put on a great show during

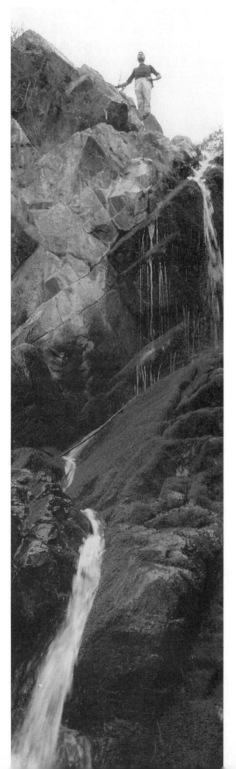
Lower falls in Hot Spring Canyon

November and December, but if the rains are late, there won't be much water cascading over the falls or flowing down the creek. Wildflowers and new leaves in early spring add to the canyon's beauty, but by then the ubiquitous poison oak bushes and vines are sporting fresh, virulent leaves, and rattlesnakes are emerging from their winter burrows. Most years, fair-weather days in January and February are best as long as you start early enough in the morning to take advantage of the limited daylight.

A portion of this route unavoidably passes through an inholding in the National Forest—the Lazy W Ranch, a church camp. You must ask for permission to hike through the property in advance. Contact the church camp, P.O. Box 579, San Juan Capistrano, CA 92675; 949-728-0141; www.lazywranch.org. The caretaker may ask that you inform someone of your safe return on your way out.

Parking is not allowed at the church camp and is very limited near the camp's entrance, so leave your car at the west end trailhead for the San Juan Trail, 0.8 mile north of Ortega Highway. Walk 0.6 mile north to the church camp entrance, then continue another 0.3 mile past several buildings. Stay close to the Hot Spring Canyon stream or streambed, and continue up an old roadbed flanked on both sides by huge, spreading coast live oak trees.

By 1.5 miles (from your car), the route deteriorates to little more than a game trail. The creek bubbles alongside, with scattered sycamores and alders growing from the granite-bouldered banks. At 2.0 miles, the canyon makes a decided turn to the northeast. From this point on, dark brownish and grayish metamorphic rocks gradually replace the granites, and the canyon becomes considerably narrower. Progress is slowed by a factor of two or three. You must choose between battling thickets of willow, sage, wild blackberry, and poison oak on the banks, or rock-hopping and sloshing through the creek while dodging nettles and alder branches. Here and there the creek may disappear under porous sands for brief stretches.

At 3.4 miles (1620´), the creek slides over a series of granite slabs and collects in limpid pools almost perennially shaded by an overhanging south wall. Fallen sycamore, oak, and alder leaves dimple the water's mirror-like surface. On the north bank, a smooth granite slab, perfect for lounging, catches early-afternoon winter sunlight; it's a nice place to rest on your return down-canyon if you have time. Just beyond, the canyon broadens, and a usually wet tributary, draining Chiquito Basin, comes in on the right. At 4.1 miles (1950´), another usually wet tributary joins on the left; a 70-foot waterfall with a scant flow lies immediately up this tributary from the main canyon.

By now, it should be possible to glimpse, just 200 yards ahead, the top of a sheer headwall. From the lip, water plunges an estimated 140 feet down two distinct tiers. Some boulder-hopping will get you to the base of a much smaller fall (a moss-covered 20-footer) just below the bottom of the big one, but further progress directly up canyon is possible only by some dicey hand-and-toe climbing.

To reach the base of the main falls, you can try backtracking a little and scrambling up the steep, broken slope to the south. As you do so, look for a raptor's aerie on a banded cliff wall to the north.

The top of the main falls can be reached by making long traverses either right or left; from there it's possible, with great effort, to continue up canyon toward the upper series of falls described in Trip 9.

Hot Spring Canyon

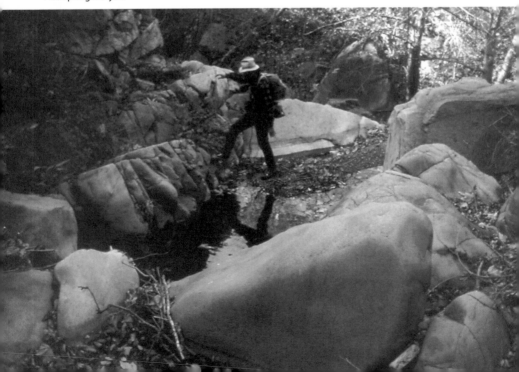

TRIP 11 Morgan Trail

Distance	5.0 miles, Point-to-point
Hiking Time	2½ hours
Elevation Gain/Loss	350'/1200'
Difficulty	Moderate
Trail Use	Dogs allowed, suitable for backpacking
Best Times	October through May
Agency	CNF/TD
Recommended Map	USFS San Mateo Canyon Wilderness topographic map
Optional Maps	USGS 7.5-min *Alberhill, Sitton Peak*
Notes	Marked trails/obvious routes, easy terrain

DIRECTIONS   EAST END: At a point on Ortega Highway 0.3 mile east of El Cariso visitor center (23 miles east of Interstate 5), drive 2.7 miles south on Killen Trail (aka South Main Divide Road) to the signed Morgan Trailhead on the right. WEST END: The trip ends at the San Juan Loop Trail parking lot, opposite the "Candy Store" on Ortega Highway, 21 miles east of Interstate 5.

As I rambled down the Morgan Trail one crisp autumn morning before dawn, the crackling of oak leaves underfoot played counterpoint to the drone of a hundred crickets singing in unison. Dozens of cold, blue stars sparkled overhead; while the moon's beams, caught in a tangled aerial net of limbs and branches, painted the ground in shades of black, gray, and silvery white. These simple kinds of sensations, jelled together, added up to a powerful, almost mystical, experience.

The Morgan Trail crosses the northern edge of San Mateo Canyon Wilderness, one of coastal Southern California's newest national-forest wilderness areas and possibly its last. You can camp overnight along portions of the trail within the wilderness boundary, but don't forget the required wilderness camping permit (see the introduction to Chapter 14 for details). This description assumes you are going to hike the trail one-way—in the north-to-south, predominantly downhill direction.

On the trail you quickly drop through manzanita and other chaparral and join the promenade of live oaks in Morrell Canyon. Willows and a few sycamores hug the canyon bottom, where water flows during the wet season. Going just this far (5 or 10 minutes in) is rewarding in itself if you have little time. At 1.0 mile

Fungus on log, Morrell Canyon

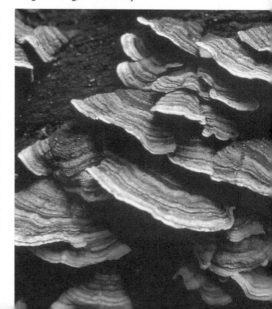

the trail cuts left (south) across the creek and rises to higher and sunnier terrain. Soon you're back on chaparral-covered slopes, dotted with granitic boulders.

At around 2.3 miles, the trail goes west along the perimeter of private lands in Potrero de la Cienaga and Round Potrero. At 2.7 miles, the trail continues west in thick chaparral. At 3.5 miles you begin a crooked descent into some oak woods, where you join the Bear Canyon Trail (4.0 miles). Stay right and continue another mile downhill through brush and boulders to the Bear Canyon trailhead adjacent to the Candy Store.

TRIP 12 Sitton Peak

Distance	9.5 miles round trip, Out-and-back
Hiking Time	5 hours (round trip)
Elevation Gain/Loss	2150'/2150'
Difficulty	Moderately strenuous
Trail Use	Dogs allowed, suitable for backpacking
Best Times	October through May
Agency	CNF/TD
Optional Map	USGS 7.5-min *Sitton Peak*
Recommended Map	USFS San Mateo Canyon Wilderness topographic map
Notes	Marked trails/obvious routes, easy terrain

DIRECTIONS Park opposite the "Candy Store" on Ortega Highway, 21 miles east of Interstate 5 at San Juan Capistrano and about 10 miles west of Lake Elsinore.

From below, Sitton Peak looks unimposing—a mere bump on a rambling ridge—despite its distinction as one of the highest points in the Santa Ana Mountains south of Ortega Highway. On the summit, though, the feeling is decidedly "top of the world." When an east or north wind blows, cleansing the sky of water vapor and air pollution, 50-mile vistas in every direction are not uncommon.

The hike to the summit is always a peaceful one, because it passes through lands included in San Mateo Canyon Wilderness. Trail camping is allowed within the wilderness area, provided you obtain the necessary free permit from the Forest Service (see introduction to Chapter 14).

Begin by taking the Bear Canyon Trail south from the Candy Store. Before long you pass into San Mateo Canyon Wilderness, where mountain bikes are banned. After 1.0 mile of moderate ascent, you come to a trail junction in the midst of a small oak woodland. Go right (as the Morgan Trail forks left) and begin climbing more steeply along a chaparral-clothed slope.

At about 1.9 miles, you reach a summit and then you descend slightly to a trail junction. You can either turn right, on an old truck trail which carries the name Bear Canyon Trail, or continue straight across on the newer and narrower Bear Ridge Trail (Bear Canyon Loop Trail on some maps). Both lead to Four Corners—originally a 4-way meeting of fire roads, and now a junction of 5 trails. The older route is more scenic, as it follows a brushy draw flanked by blue-flowering ceanothus, and visits Pigeon Spring, with an old watering trough and the last bit of shade you may find on the way to the peak.

At Four Corners, swing right on the wide path climbing northwest—a disused section of the Sitton Peak Road. After a steady ascent of about 300 vertical feet, you reach a flat area (4.0 miles) just below a boulder-studded ridge, with a 3250-foot high point, to the north. Easily climbed, the ridge summit offers a view somewhat similar to that seen from Sitton Peak. The flat area by the road (just inside the wilderness boundary) makes a

good overnight campsite for those who backpack in.

Beyond the flat area the road descends another 0.5 mile to a saddle just below Sitton Peak. From this saddle, you leave the road and follow a steep, informal trail up through scattered manzanita and chamise on the east slope of the peak.

The view from the top is especially impressive to the west. Here the foothills and western canyons of the Santa Anas merge with the creeping suburbs of southern Orange County. Beyond lies the flat, blue ocean punctuated by the profile of Santa Catalina Island. Some 2000 feet below, toylike cars on the highway make their way down the sinuous course of San Juan Canyon.

TRIP 13 Lucas Canyon

Distance	14 miles, Point-to-point
Hiking Time	7 hours
Elevation Gain/Loss	2000'/3200'
Difficulty	Strenuous
Trail Use	Dogs allowed, suitable for backpacking
Best Times	November through May
Agency	CNF/TD
Optional Maps	USGS 7.5-min *Sitton Peak, Canada Gobernadora*
Recommended Map	USFS San Mateo Canyon Wilderness topographic map
Notes	Marked trails/obvious routes, bushwhacking, moderate terrain

DIRECTIONS EAST END: Park opposite the "Candy Store" on Ortega Highway, 21 miles east of Interstate 5 at San Juan Capistrano and about 10 miles west of Lake Elsinore. WEST END: The trip ends at a point on Ortega Highway just west of Hot Springs Canyon Road, 12.5 miles east of Interstate 5.

Under construction for years, primarily through the efforts of volunteer workers, the Lucas Canyon Trail was finally completed in 1992. The opening of the trail inaugurated the first legal access to the San Mateo Canyon Wilderness trail system from the west. Shortly

thereafter, in October 1993, virtually all of the vegetation traversed by the trail was incinerated to ash and blackened twigs when flames swept through.

In all the years since, the regrowth of vegetation has been rapid, and the trail has received spotty maintenance, again by volunteers. What this means is that some sections are likely to be rough and possibly overgrown at various times. Also, as of this writing, there are questions about private-property infringement on the lower end of the trail. Check with the Forest Service first if you are planning a trip on this trail, and failing that, a query to Caspers Wilderness Park may help.

Lucas Canyon has been called Orange County's "Mother Lode"—an overstated reference to the placer mining activity that took place here in the late 1800s. If you see old mining debris in the canyon, remember that it is considered "historical" and therefore must be left as is.

Begin, as in Trip 12 above, by following the Bear Canyon Trail south to the Four Corners trail junction, 3.2 miles. From there, take the Verdugo Trail (old Verdugo Truck Trail) southwest across dry, chaparral-coated hillsides. At 5.8 miles, the Bluewater Trail intersects on the left. Keep straight and bend right (west) through a shady oak woodland to the next trail junction (6.3 miles), just north of a rounded 2616-foot hill. Here, turn right and head north on the Lucas Canyon Trail.

Nearly 3 miles of sometimes-steep descent lie ahead. To the south, you may spot some houses on the nearby ridgeline; these are part of the Rancho Carrillo development—an inholding in the wilderness area. After a long mile, these signs of civilization disappear as you descend on switchbacks over rough, rocky terrain. The bottom of Lucas Canyon, a steep gorge at this point, lies to your left. You cross the stream in the bottom of this gorge at 8.5 miles, traverse for a while along the south wall of the gorge, and descend again to the stream, which in this area flows about half the year. For the next 1.5 miles, the trail sticks close to the stream, and you may see evidence hereabouts of past gold-mining.

At 10.0 miles, the trail leaves the stream, bending northward along a small tributary toward the ridge above. At 11.5 miles you strike that ridge and turn right on an old truck trail. This brings you to Sitton Peak Road in less than half a mile. Turn left there and make a winding, nearly 2-mile descent to Ortega Highway. Turn right and walk 0.25 mile along the highway to San Juan Fire Station, the nearest available parking spot.

Chapter 14

Santa Ana Mountains—
San Mateo Canyon Wilderness

Down along the creek, a warm breeze carries the scent of sage and blooming chaparral. There's no sound but the distant drone of bees, the soft music of water coursing down polished rock, and your own footsteps. A fat gopher snake lounging by the creek stiffens at your approach. Tiny fish dart about in the stream eddies, while a pond turtle launches itself from a rock shelf, deftly slicing through the surface of a crystalline pool. You might as well be a thousand miles away from civilization.

This is the world of San Mateo Canyon, the heart of one of California's few coastal wilderness areas, the 62-square-mile San Mateo Canyon Wilderness. Carved out of the southernmost one-third of the Cleveland National Forest's Trabuco District, this charming but rugged area lies within 30 airline miles of 6 million people. Only 10 miles away are the expanding edges of three of the nation's fastest-growing suburban regions: southern Orange County, southwestern Riverside County, and northern San Diego County.

San Mateo Canyon may seem a short distance away by the map, but getting there may prove problematic. Some access roads receive little maintenance and may become impassable in wet weather. Exploring the inner sanctum of

the wilderness can be both physically taxing and mentally stimulating; trails may melt into the scenery, and you can lose track of your position. But these difficulties are exactly what shields the area from casual users. If you're willing to put up with them, this is your paradise.

Prepare to make a long day of it, or pack in enough equipment to stay a night or two along the trail. Unlike many national-forest wilderness areas in California, which require wilderness permits for both day and overnight use, this one requires a permit only for overnight use (backpacking). Camping regulations emphasize the importance of fire control. Campfires are never allowed within the wilderness, though backpacking stoves are permitted if used within areas cleared of flammable vegetation. No mountain bikes are allowed either, in accordance with a general prohibition of mechanical conveyances—even wheeled carts—in all federal wilderness areas.

Wilderness camping permits can be obtained at the El Cariso visitor center at El Cariso Station on Ortega Highway, and at any Cleveland National Forest fire or ranger station. Since many of the ranger and fire stations keep irregular hours during the rainy months, it may be best to apply well in advance by mail or phone to the Trabuco Ranger District office in

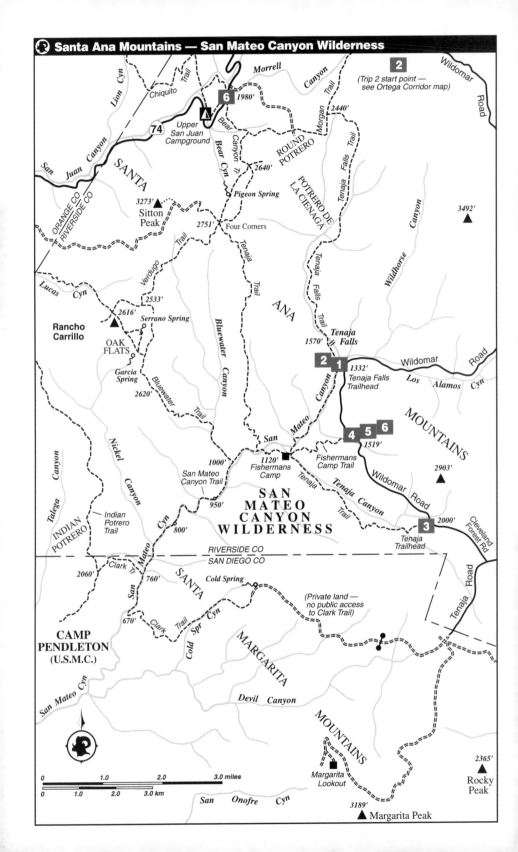

Santa Ana Mountains — San Mateo Canyon Wilderness

2 (Trip 2 start point — see Ortega Corridor map)

Morrell Canyon

Wildomar Road

6 1980'

Upper San Juan Campground

74

Chiquito Trail

Lion Cyn

San Juan Canyon

Bear Canyon Tr

Bear Cyn

2640'

Pigeon Spring

2440'

Morgan Trail

ROUND POTRERO

POTRERO DE LA CIENAGA

Tenaja Falls Trail

3492'

ORANGE CO RIVERSIDE CO

SANTA

3273'
Sitton Peak

2751' Four Corners

Verdugo Trail

Tenaja Trail

Wildhorse Canyon

Lucas Cyn

2533'

ANA

Rancho Carrillo

2616'
Serrano Spring

OAK FLATS

Garcia Spring

2620'

Bluewater Canyon

Bluewater Trail

Tenaja Falls Trail

1570' Tenaja Falls

2 **1** 1332'
Tenaja Falls Trailhead

Wildomar Road

Los Alamos Cyn

MOUNTAINS

San Mateo Canyon

4 **5** **6**
1519'

Fishermans Camp Trail

2903'

Nickel Canyon

San Mateo Canyon Trail

1000'

1120'
Fishermans Camp

950'

SAN
MATEO
CANYON
WILDERNESS

Tenaja Canyon

Tenaja Trail

Wildomar Road

3 2000'
Tenaja Trailhead

Cleveland Forest Rd

Talega Canyon

Indian Potrero Trail

INDIAN POTRERO

San Mateo Cyn

800'

RIVERSIDE CO
SAN DIEGO CO

2060'

Clark Tr

760'

Cold Spring

Cold Spr Cyn

SANTA

Clark Tr

Cold Spr Cyn

Clark Trail

670'

Clark Trail

Cold Spr Cyn

(Private land — no public access to Clark Trail)

Tenaja Road

CAMP
PENDLETON
(U.S.M.C.)

San Mateo Cyn

MARGARITA

Devil Canyon

MOUNTAINS

2365'

Margarita Lookout

Rocky Peak

San Onofre Cyn

3189' ▲ Margarita Peak

| 0 | 1.0 | 2.0 | 3.0 miles |
| 0 | 1.0 | 2.0 | 3.0 km |

Corona (see Appendix 5). The Corona office is also your best source for information about national-forest road conditions.

Three primary entrance points have been designated for San Mateo Canyon Wilderness. The northern two are the San Juan Loop Trail trailhead, across from the Candy Store on Ortega Highway, and the Morgan Trailhead on Killen Trail, or South Main Divide Road. This book's Chapter 13, Ortega Corridor map, page 152, shows these entrances best.

The primary entrance to the south half of the wilderness is the Tenaja Trailhead, accessible via Murrieta in southwestern Riverside County. From most parts of Orange County, it takes 80 or 90 minutes to get there. Drive south on Interstate 15 from Corona and exit at Clinton Keith Road. Proceed 5 miles south on Clinton Keith Road (passing through the Santa Rosa Plateau Ecological Reserve), and curve sharply right where the road becomes Tenaja Road. After 1.7 more miles make a right turn to

remain on Tenaja Road. Continue west on Tenaja Road for another 4.2 miles, then go right on the one-lane, paved Cleveland Forest Road. Proceed another mile to the trailhead parking area, which features restrooms and well water delivered by a hand pump.

Heading north from the Tenaja Trailhead by car, you can follow the narrow, paved Wildomar Road, which replaces the former dirt road called Tenaja Truck Trail on older maps, down to secondary trailheads (basically turnouts or small parking lots) at Fishermans Camp Trail (for Trips 4, 5, and 6 in this section) and at Tenaja Falls Trail. Beyond the Tenaja Falls trailhead, Wildomar Road, paved all the way now, reaches the Wildomar Off-Road Vehicle Area, and continues north to Ortega Highway as Killen Trail (South Main Divide Road). Note that Wildomar Road, particularly between Widomar ORV area and Tenaja Trailhead, is subject to vehicle closure due to wet weather in winter or hazardous fire conditions in summer.

Hiking San Mateo Canyon

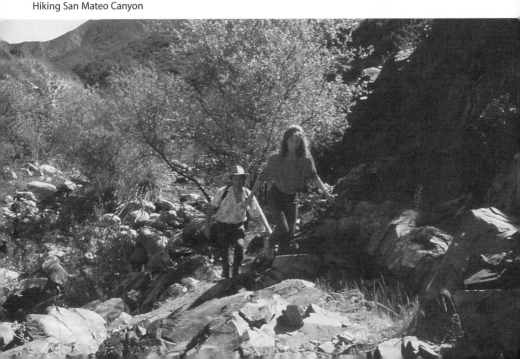

The forest service has published an up-to-date (2003) topographic map of San Mateo Canyon Wilderness (with the neighboring Agua Tibia Wilderness in Riverside and San Diego counties on the reverse side). Although the contour-interval on this map is 80 feet—not as fine as the 40-foot contours on the USGS 7.5-minute topo maps—and some of the trail alignments are only approximately shown, this is the best map to have for any exploration of San Mateo Canyon Wilderness and adjoining national forest areas south of Ortega Highway.

TRIP 1 Tenaja Falls

Distance	1.4 miles round trip, Out-and-back
Hiking Time	1 hour (round trip)
Elevation Gain/Loss	300'/300'
Difficulty	Easy
Trail Use	Dogs allowed, good for kids, suitable for backpacking
Best Times	December through June
Agency	CNF/TD
Recommended Map	USFS San Mateo Canyon Wilderness topographic map
Optional Map	USGS 7.5-min *Sitton Peak*
Notes	Marked trails/obvious routes, easy terrain

DIRECTIONS Exit Interstate 15 at Clinton Keith Road in Murrieta. Proceed 5 miles south on Clinton Keith Road (passing into the Santa Rosa Plateau Ecological Reserve), and curve sharply right where the road becomes Tenaja Road. After 1.7 more miles make a right turn to remain on Tenaja Road. Continue west on Tenaja Road for another 4.2 miles, then go right on the one-lane, paved Cleveland Forest Road. Proceed another mile to the Tenaja Trailhead. Continue another 4.3 miles north on the narrow pavement of Wildomar Road (formerly Old Tenaja Road) to the Tenaja Falls Trail parking area on the left.

With five tiers and a total drop of about 150 feet, Tenaja Falls is the most interesting natural feature in San Mateo Canyon Wilderness. In late winter and spring, water coursing down the polished rock produces a kind of soothing music not widely heard in this somewhat dry corner of the Santa Ana Mountains.

On foot, head downhill to San Mateo Creek and cross it on the concrete ford of an old roadbed. Make certain you cross that creek first. If you bear right too soon you will be following another stream going through Los Alamos Canyon—an easy mistake.

You might have to wade through an ankle-deep or greater flow to get across San Mateo Creek. Continue north on the steadily rising former fire road and you'll soon be treated to a fairly distant view of the falls. After 0.7 mile the road passes near the upper lip of the falls, where a few large oaks provide welcome shade.

Further close exploration of the falls requires rock-climbing skills and extreme caution. The flow of water has worn the granitic rock almost glassy smooth. Don't be lured into dangerous situations. A somewhat safer way of approaching the lower falls is to scramble over the rough-textured rocks well away from the water. You could also backtrack down the road and then scramble down the slope into the brush-choked creekbed down near the base of the falls.

Upper tier, Tenaja Falls

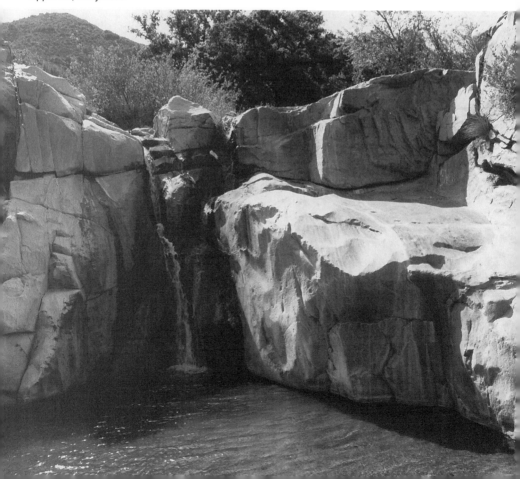

TRIP 2 Tenaja Falls Traverse

Distance	8.2 miles, Point-to-point
Hiking Time	4 hours
Elevation Gain/Loss	600'/1450'
Difficulty	Moderately strenuous
Trail Use	Dogs allowed, suitable for backpacking
Best Times	November through May
Agency	CNF/TD
Recommended Map	USFS San Mateo Canyon Wilderness topographic map
Optional Maps	USGS 7.5-min *Alberhill, Sitton Peak*
Notes	Marked trails/obvious routes, easy terrain

DIRECTIONS NORTH END: At a point on Ortega Highway 0.3 mile east of El Cariso visitor center (23 miles east of Interstate 5), drive 2.7 miles south on Killen Trail (aka South Main Divide Road) to the signed Morgan Trailhead on the right. SOUTH END: The hike ends at the Tenaja Falls Trail parking area on the west side of Wildomar Road, 14 miles south of the Morgan Trailhead by way of Killen Trail and Wildomar Road.

The one-way traverse from the Morgan Trailhead on the South Main Divide down to the Tenaja Falls trailhead in San Mateo Canyon lets you see plenty of gorgeous springtime scenery—without repeating any steps. You can set up a car-shuttle arrangement, or have someone drop you off at the start and later pick you up at the finish. Or, with just one car, you might think of a way to use a bicycle (to be left at the start or end point) to turn this trek into a hybrid hike/bike loop. Bikes are not allowed on the hiking route itself, but they are well suited to traveling the 14 miles of mostly narrow, thinly paved Wildomar Road connecting the start and finish points of the hike.

From Morgan Trailhead you begin with a short descent through chaparral on the Morgan Trail. Soon, you enter the boundary of San Mateo Canyon Wilderness and plunge into the dark, upper reaches of Morrell Canyon. The canyon is loaded with magnificent live oaks, the ever-hardy survivors of periodic wildfires. The trail crosses Morrell Canyon's

small creek at 1.0 mile, then rises back into the sunny chaparral.

At 2.2 miles, Tenaja Falls Trail branches left. Heading east, you cross a wooded ravine and steadily and crookedly rise on rocky, chaparral-clad slopes. Later you turn south on those slopes, still climbing, and skirt the boundary of a parcel of private land lying within both the national forest and the wilderness area. Most of this private inholding covers the flat, grassy valley named Potrero de la Cienega (translation: "Pasture of the Marsh."), which sheds its water into upper San Mateo Canyon.

Mariposa lily along Tenaja Falls Trail

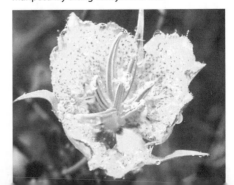

Climbing ends at a high point just above the 2800-foot contour, some 400 feet above flat floor of the potrero. You then descend south into the southeastern corner of the potrero. At 4.3 miles you join a disused dirt road, which continues going south around the east edge of the potrero. In the next mile, there are plenty of potential backpacking campsites amid scattered live oaks.

The old road curls west around the inholding and then, starting at 5.5 miles, assumes a descending course south down the left side of V-shaped upper San Mateo Canyon. You can often hear water cascading down the canyon bottom, which is virtually impossible to reach due to dense chaparral growth.

By 7.0 miles you're right alongside the canyon bottom, and you benefit from the soothing sound of rushing water and the sheltering shade of streamside oaks. At 7.5 miles you cross San Mateo Canyon's creek on an old concrete ford just above Tenaja Falls, switching over to the canyon's west side. After rapidly descending on the popular southernmost leg of Tenaja Falls Trail, there's only one more creek crossing to contend with, plus a short climb up to the Teneja Falls trailhead.

TRIP 3 Tenaja Canyon

Distance	7.4 miles (to Fishermans Camp and back), Out-and-back
Hiking Time	3½ hours (round trip)
Elevation Gain/Loss	1300'/1300'
Difficulty	Moderately strenuous
Trail Use	Dogs allowed, suitable for backpacking, good for kids
Best Times	November through May
Agency	CNF/TD
Recommended Map	USFS San Mateo Canyon Wilderness topographic map
Optional Maps	USGS 7.5-min *Wildomar, Sitton Peak*
Notes	Marked trails/obvious routes, easy terrain

DIRECTIONS Exit Interstate 15 at Clinton Keith Road in Murrieta. Proceed 5 miles south on Clinton Keith Road (passing into the Santa Rosa Plateau Ecological Reserve), and curve sharply right where the road becomes Tenaja Road. After 1.7 more miles make a right turn to remain on Tenaja Road. Continue west on Tenaja Road for another 4.2 miles, then go right on the one-lane, paved Cleveland Forest Road. Proceed another mile to the Tenaja Trailhead.

A s the gloom of a late afternoon descended upon the deep-cut, linear furrow of Tenaja Canyon, dozens of orange-bellied newts waddled determinedly uphill and across the trail, oblivious to my footfalls. The cute faces and beady eyes of these little amphibians mirrored a mindless desire I could not fathom: sex in a bower of leaf litter and ferns? A bellyful of succulent tree-dwelling insects, ripe for the taking?

The south segment of the Tenaja Trail follows Tenaja Canyon down to its confluence with San Mateo Canyon. Unlike all other hikes in this book, the route takes you down and later all the way back up, so remember that if the day is warm or you feel fatigued, you can always reverse your course at any time.

At the start, Tenaja Trailhead, an old-fashioned hand pump dispenses cold, sweet water. Post your adventure pass on your car, and head downhill on the trail going west. A few minutes' descent takes you to the shady bowels of V-shaped Tenaja Canyon, where huge coast live oaks and pale-barked sycamores frame a limpid, rock-dimpled stream. Mostly the trail ahead meanders alongside the

Coast range newt

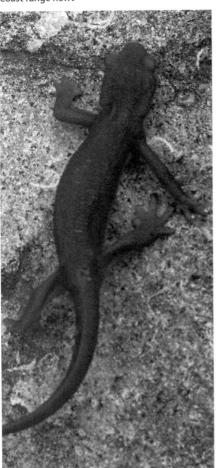

stream, but for the canyon's middle stretch it carves its way across the chaparral-blanketed south wall, 200–400 feet above the canyon bottom.

After 3.7 miles of general descent, you reach Fishermans Camp, a former drive-in campground at one time accessible by many miles of bad road. Today the site, distinguished by its parklike setting amid a live oak grove, serves as a fine wilderness campsite for an overnight backpack trip (a wilderness permit is required for this). The name of the place hints of the fishing opportunities afforded by nearby San Mateo Canyon creek during and after the rainy season. A native species of steelhead trout was recently discovered in this drainage, surprising experts who thought that steelhead might be extinct south of Los Angeles County.

At Fishermans Camp, three other trails diverge. Fishermans Camp Trail (the abandoned road to the former camp) travels east uphill to Old Tenaja Road. The San Mateo Trail, a narrow footpath, continues northeast up San Mateo Canyon to the Tenaja Falls Trailhead. To the west, the San Mateo Trail heads down San Mateo Canyon and connects with the northern segment of the Tenaja Trail, which goes to Four Corners and Bear Canyon Trail.

TRIP 4 Fishermans Camp Loop

Distance	5.0 miles, Loop
Hiking Time	2½ hours
Elevation Gain/Loss	550'/550'
Difficulty	Moderate
Trail Use	Dogs allowed, suitable for backpacking, good for kids
Best Times	November through May
Agency	CNF/TD
Recommended Map	USFS San Mateo Canyon Wilderness topographic map
Optional Map	USGS 7.5-min *Sitton Peak*
Notes	Marked trails/obvious routes, easy terrain

Santa Ana Mountains
San Mateo Canyon

DIRECTIONS Exit Interstate 15 at Clinton Keith Road in Murrieta. Proceed 5 miles south on Clinton Keith Road (passing into the Santa Rosa Plateau Ecological Reserve), and curve sharply right where the road becomes Tenaja Road. After 1.7 more miles make a right turn to remain on Tenaja Road. Continue west on Tenaja Road for another 4.2 miles, then go right on the one-lane, paved Cleveland Forest Road. Proceed another mile to the Tenaja Trailhead. Continue another 2.7 miles north on the narrow pavement of Wildomar Road (formerly Old Tenaja Road) to reach the small parking turnout for Fishermans Camp Trail on the left.

After a good rain, upper San Mateo Canyon brims with cold, sparkling water. If you come on a sunny winter day, you can often enjoy a couple of hours of very comfortable, almost summer-like temperatures. By midafternoon low sunlight floods the canyon, and you may be tempted to slide into one of the shallow pools for a quick cooling-off.

From the parking turnout, an old road, reverted to a hiking trail called Fishermans Camp Trail, descends to the abandoned Fishermans Camp, a former drive-in campground, 1.5 miles away. The camp lies at the mouth of Tenaja Canyon, whose linear alignment is associated with a rift called the Tenaja Fault.

Beautifully shaded by oaks and sycamores, Fishermans Camp is an idyllic and practical setting for a trail camp. Camp stoves can be used in one of the large bare patches amid the knee-high grass (remember, though, no campfires

are allowed). In winter and spring water in Tenaja Canyon's stream trickles by on its way to the bottom of San Mateo Canyon, just 300 yards north.

A restful pause at this seductive spot is alone worth the trip, but there's more to see ahead. Find the narrow trail going north (just east of the brook in Tenaja Canyon) toward boulder-strewn, vegetation-choked San Mateo Canyon. There you will cross the creek and swing north to follow the canyon upstream along the canyon's west side. You curve around the mouth of a prominent side canyon, and then go across a grassy bench. Ahead lie three more creek crossings and a couple of passages through live oaks and chaparral. Several shallow pools, set amid colorful metamorphic slabs in the canyon bottom, may tempt you into trying a cooling dip. Spring wildflowers include bush lupine, snapdragon penstemon, monkeyflowers of various hues, owl's

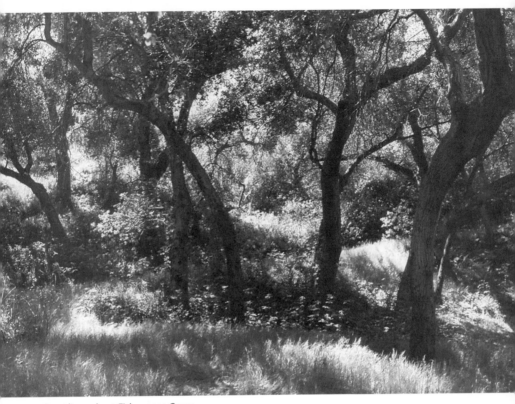

Coast live oaks at Fishermans Camp

clover, paintbrush, and wild morning glory. Yuccas send up their candle-like flower stalks along the hillsides.

After the fourth creek crossing, the trail sticks to the right bank until, 1.9 miles from Fisherman's Camp, you arrive at the Tenaja Falls trailhead along Wildomar Road. Close the loop by walking 1.5 miles on Wildomar Road back to your car.

TRIP 5 San Mateo Canyon

Distance	7.0 miles (to Lunch Rock and back), Out-and-back
Hiking Time	4 hours (round trip)
Elevation Gain/Loss	800'/800'
Difficulty	Moderately strenuous
Trail Use	Dogs allowed, suitable for backpacking
Best Times	November through May
Agency	CNF/TD
Recommended Map	USFS San Mateo Canyon Wilderness topographic map
Optional Map	USGS 7.5-min *Sitton Peak*
Notes	Marked trails/obvious routes, moderate terrain

DIRECTIONS Exit Interstate 15 at Clinton Keith Road in Murrieta. Proceed 5 miles south on Clinton Keith Road (passing into the Santa Rosa Plateau Ecological Reserve), and curve sharply right where the road becomes Tenaja Road. After 1.7 more miles make a right turn to remain on Tenaja Road. Continue west on Tenaja Road for another 4.2 miles, then go right on the one-lane, paved Cleveland Forest Road. Proceed another mile to the Tenaja Trailhead. Continue another 2.7 miles north on the narrow pavement of Wildomar Road (formerly Old Tenaja Road) to reach the small parking turnout for Fishermans Camp Trail on the left.

With no roads and sometimes only the barest hint of a trail in view, San Mateo Canyon's inner depths are the essence of wilderness. The sky above is bluest blue, and the air is alive with moist, woodsy odors. The canyon walls resonate with gurgling water. Papery sycamore leaves chafe on the wind, and birds flit noisily about, staking out territory in brush and tree tops. Under the shade of live oaks, Indian morteros pock a granite slab. In the stream below, pond turtles hitching rides on the current careen from rock to rock. A gopher snake on the bank slithers through dry grass in search of a small, furry meal. Only the passing of high-flying aircraft gives evidence of the outside world a few miles away.

Following the canyon may be a bit problematic. You'll be tracing the latest incarnation of the San Mateo Canyon Trail, originally constructed before the turn of the century. Trail maintenance is occasional. Floods routinely obliterate the trail where it passes close to the creekbed, and rapid regeneration of riparian vegetation and grasses tends to conceal what remains. Poison oak, nettles, and other irritating plants abound along the streambed, so wear long pants in these areas.

Begin, as in Trip 4 above, by descending to Fishermans Camp at the mouth of Tenaja Canyon. This is the site of one of several primitive fishing camps that lined San Mateo Canyon before World War II. During a series of wet winters in the 1930s, steelhead (sea-running rainbow trout) ran upstream to spawn in San Mateo Canyon's middle and upper reaches. More runs occurred in 1969, and again during the late 1990s.

From the west edge of the grassy, oak-bowered clearing at Fishermans Camp, find the foot trail through ceanothus and scrub oak that rises onto the south wall of

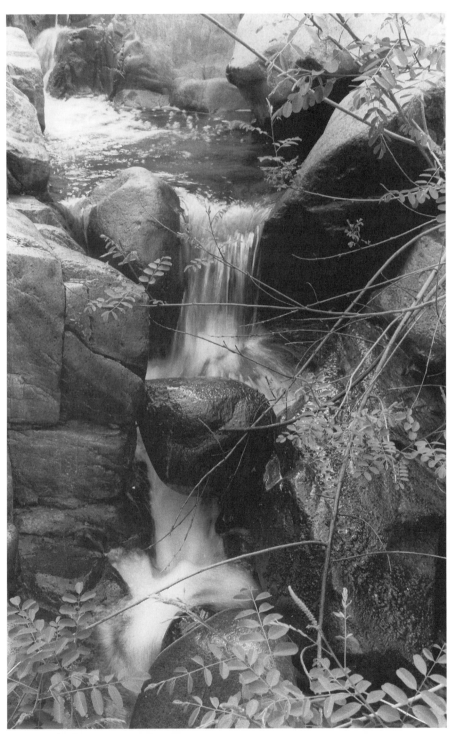

San Mateo Creek

San Mateo Canyon. This part of the trail avoids a narrow, vegetation-choked section of the canyon about 200 feet below. After 0.4 mile you round a bend and drop quickly down 10 switchbacks to the bottom of San Mateo Canyon. Next you face a 200-yard passage through a veritable jungle of ferns, poison oak, and wild berry vines. After that you come to a creek crossing. Wade through, or skip across on the stones. From now on stay on the right (north) bank as you continue downstream.

The next quarter mile or so of trail may be washed out. An easy scramble gets you over a low outcropping of crumbling metamorphic rock on the right. Then, as the canyon widens, the trail diverges from the stream a little and traverses an oak-dotted potrero ("pasture," or grassy area). About 0.5 mile past the creek crossing, the trail dips to cross two shallow stream bottoms (usually dry) just below the mouth of Bluewater Canyon. Just beyond the second wash is a signed junction with the Bluewater Trail. Stay left and continue down San Mateo Canyon. Another 0.7 mile ahead, the canyon bottom narrows and the water slides over car-sized boulders and gathers in languid pools (950′ elevation). About 50 square miles of watershed lie upstream of this point. A large flat-topped rock, dubbed "Lunch Rock" by hikers, overlooks the stream here. A newer stretch of trail on the right bypasses Lunch Rock, but you can stay down along the stream to reach the rock itself. You've come 3.5 miles from the starting point, probably the farthest you would want to venture in a single day. After sunning, swimming, eating, and a siesta, it's uphill all the way back.

For backpackers, San Mateo Canyon offers a number of pleasant campsites. Dry, sandy benches along the wider parts of the canyon abound. Any such campsite could be used as a base camp for further dayhike explorations. The following is a description of what lies beyond Lunch Rock.

Down-canyon from Lunch Rock, travel may be impeded in places by big boulders and dense growths of cattails, wild grape vines, blackberry vines, stinging nettles, mulefat, and willow saplings. If the existing trail leads into impenetrable brush thickets, then try wading the creek. At the 800-foot contour (4.7 miles from Wildomar Road), there's a fine swimming hole, about 5 feet deep, set amid outcrops of dark gray metamorphic rock. Near Nickel Canyon, 5.3 miles, your speed may increase as you pick up the bed of an old mining road.

At 5.9 miles you reach a junction with the west branch of the Clark Trail, more recently called the Indian Potrero Trail. A side trip up this trail (a gain of 1300 feet in 1.3 miles) would take you to Indian Potrero, a bald area on the north ridge overlooking San Mateo Canyon. The other roads and trails to Indian Potrero come from access-restricted Camp Pendleton or from private lands having no public access.

For a mile further the trail continues down San Mateo Canyon along the bed of the old mining road, where you can spot evidence of the mining days—old rusted equipment and a tumbledown hut—in the shade of the oaks. Then comes Clark Trail rising on the left, a so-called land-locked route that currently has no exit on public land and receives scant maintenance. Beyond the Clark Trail junction lies a trail-less passage down through the most beautiful part of San Mateo Canyon, where the creek dances over sun-warmed granite and swirls through shallow pools. At a point 2 miles down from Clark Trail, the creek enters Camp Pendleton, where entry is prohibited.

TRIP 6 Bluewater Traverse

Distance	12.7 miles, Point-to-point
Hiking Time	7 hours
Elevation Gain/Loss	2450'/2900'
Difficulty	Strenuous
Trail Use	Dogs allowed, suitable for backpacking
Best Times	November through May
Agency	CNF/TD
Recommended Map	USFS San Mateo Canyon Wilderness topographic map
Optional Map	USGS 7.5-min *Sitton Peak*
Notes	Navigation required, bushwhacking, moderate terrain

DIRECTIONS NORTH END: Begin opposite the "Candy Store" on Ortega Highway, 21 miles east of Interstate 5 at San Juan Capistrano and about 10 miles west of Lake Elsinore. SOUTH END: The hike ends at the top of the Fishermans Camp Trail, 2.7 miles north of the Teneja Trailhead and 1.6 miles south of the Tenaja Falls Trail parking area.

From Ortega Highway on the north to Tenaja Road on the south, this route traverses the heart of the San Mateo Wilderness by way of old roads and primitive trails. Carry a full backpack and plan to spend a night out in Oak Flats or San Mateo Canyon, or go light and make this simply a long day's outing. Without a doubt, March and April are the most rewarding times: knee-high grasses ripple across the potreros, chaparral blooms release their potent fragrances, and water trickles down the shady ravines. Depending on its state of maintenance, the Bluewater Trail may be quite overgrown by encroaching vegetation, so it would be wise to contact the Forest Service before attempting this route.

From the Candy Store on Ortega Highway, follow the Bear Canyon Trail (see Chapter 13, Trip 12) south to Four Corners, 3.2 miles. From Four Corners there are two routes leading into San Mateo Canyon. On the left (southeast) is the north branch of the Tenaja Trail, monotonously following the spine of a treeless ridge all the way to the canyon.

Our way, the Verdugo Trail straight ahead (southwest), is much more interesting.

For a mile or so the Verdugo Trail winds along steep, brushy slopes offering excellent views of the San Mateo Canyon drainage and the rounded Santa Margarita Mountains to the south. Passing over the shoulder of a ridge, the roadbed suddenly drops about 400 feet to cross an oak-shaded tributary of Bluewater Canyon (4.7 miles). Winding upward, then down again you reach, around 5.5 miles, the edge of a pleasant woodland—several hundred rolling acres shaded by live oaks and tall chaparral. At 5.8 miles, bear left and follow the Bluewater Trail east and south past Serrano Spring and Garcia Spring in the Oak Flats area.

Oak Flats is one of the nicest back corners of the Trabuco District, containing a charming mixture of oak-rimmed potreros and deeply shaded ravines. Until fairly recently, some Scottish Highlander cattle used these meadows as grazing grounds. Meadow wildflowers include owl's clover, lupine, blue-eyed grass, and some non-natives typically found in formerly grazed areas: filaree and scarlet pimpernel.

A complete reconnaissance of the Oak Flats area might include a visit to nearby peak 2616, overlooking the private Rancho Carrillo development in Verdugo Potrero (an area well within the overall outlines of, but excluded from San Mateo Canyon Wilderness by a "cherry-stem" boundary). The coastline is only 13 air-miles away from here, and the wide, blue arc of the Pacific Ocean can be seen on most days.

During winter and spring, water trickles down the ravine containing Serrano and Garcia springs, and flows onward toward Nickel Canyon. With purification, it can be used by backpackers camping overnight in the area.

Beyond Oak Flats, the poor roadbed that has so far served as the Bluewater Trail veers left (southeast) and attains a nearly barren summit (7.5 miles). After about 250 yards, the roadbed turns southwest, while the Bluewater Trail (a footpath) continues southeast, descending gradually toward Bluewater Canyon, 1500 feet below. After a short, confusing stretch through a grassy area, the route pitches very sharply downward down a brushy ridgeline. Newer switchbacks do little to keep the feet from sliding; backpackers may at times feel safer sliding down on the seat of the pants! There's a short respite about halfway down, followed by gentler switchbacks down to the bottom of the canyon (9.0 miles).

After the effort of descent, the cold, bubbling stream in Bluewater Canyon is the hiker's equivalent of paradise. Small oaks and sycamores provide semi-shade. The Bluewater Trail, overgrown by small shrubs and grasses, continues downstream on the banks for 0.8 mile, crossing the creek several times.

Don't miss the obscure junction with the San Mateo Canyon Trail on a bench at Bluewater Canyon's mouth (9.8 miles). Turn left here and work your way east along the left side of San Mateo Canyon. Just beyond the creek crossing (10.5 miles) pick up the series of switchbacks leading toward Fishermans Camp. Wildomar Road is 1.5 miles beyond that by way of the Fishermans Camp Trail.

Opposite the creek crossing, on the nose of a long ridge leading north, you'll spot the switchbacks of the north branch of Tenaja Trail, which leads back to Four Corners. If you want to loop back to Ortega Highway, this is the expedient if tedious way to go.

Whipple yucca along Verdugo Trail

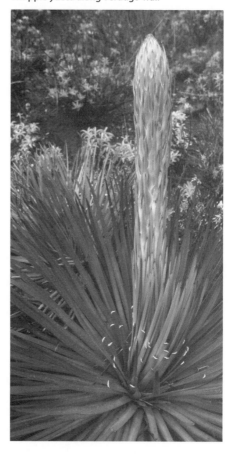

Appendix 1
Best Hikes

Best Beach Hike
San Onofre State Beach (Chapter 5, Trip 3). Here the primeval Southern California coastline survives more or less intact.

Best Suburban Hikes
El Moro Canyon Loop (Chapter 3, Trip 4). Ocean views and passages through dark, spooky oak groves.

Laurel Canyon Loop (Chapter 4, Trip 3). A still-wild coastal canyon with oaks, sycamores, and a seasonal waterfall.

Telegraph Canyon Traverse (Chapter 6, Trip 8). Oak-dotted hills and gentle canyons.

Oak Canyon Nature Center (Chapter 7, Trip 1). An agreeable patch of wilderness amidst the wilds of suburban Anaheim.

Borrego Canyon to Red Rock (Chapter 8, Trip 1). Shady canyon and eroded sandstone cliffs.

Best Mountain Hikes
Holy Jim Falls (Chapter 12, Trip 11). An intimate canyon setting highlighted by a picturesque little waterfall.

West Horsethief-Trabuco Canyon Loop (Chapter 12, Trip 15). From shady canyon to viewful summit ridge, and back down.

Best Canyon Hikes
Harding Canyon (Chapter 12, Trip 9). Narrow, rugged, sublime canyon graced with a crystal-clear winter-time stream.

San Mateo Canyon (Chapter 14, Trips 4 and 5). Ramble among oaks, wildflowers, and pools along San Mateo Creek.

Best Waterfalls
Ortega Falls (Chapter 13, Trip 2). Short hike from Ortega Highway. Impressive in wet years.

Lower Hot Spring Canyon (Chapter 13, Trip 10). Water falls 140 feet—Orange County's tallest. Remote, difficult; inaccessible to the average hiker.

Tenaja Falls (Chapter 14, Trip 1). A multitiered cascade hewn in polished granite. Easy hike to get there.

Best View Hikes
Emerald Vista Point (Chapter 3, Trip 3). Bird's-eye view of Orange County's coast and the offshore islands.

Laguna Bowl Loop (Chapter 4, Trip 7). Long views of the Laguna Beach coastline and interior mountains.

Santiago Peak (Chapter 12, Trip 12). 100-mile views encompassing most of coastal southern California.

Best Wildflowers

Los Santos-Trans Preserve Loop (Chapter 11, Trip 5). Catch some of California's finest springtime displays of greenery and wildflowers in March or April.

San Juan Loop Trail (Chapter 13, Trip 3). Wildflowers of the mountain meadows and chaparral.

Bluewater Traverse (Chapter 14, Trip 6). Wildflowers of the chaparral and potrero country.

Best Autumn Colors

Trabuco Canyon (Chapter 12, Trip 14). Tawny colors of willow, sycamore, and maple. Best in December.

Best Bird and Wildlife Watching

San Joaquin Wildlife Sanctuary (Chapter 2, Trip 2). Local as well as migrant bird life.

Bell Canyon (Chapter 10, Trips 2–4). Frequented by deer, bobcats, and mountain lions.

Chiquito Basin (Chapter 13, Trip 5). A sunny, oak-rimmed valley; a natural pasture.

San Mateo Canyon (Chapter 14, all trips). Aquatic, oak woodland, and chaparral habitats attract a wide variety of reptiles, amphibians, birds and mammals.

Best Mountain Biking and Running Trails

Crystal Cove backcountry area (Chapter 3, Trips 3, 4, and 5). The entire backcountry part of the state park is mountain-bike friendly. A variety of challenging fire roads and single-track trails.

Aliso and Wood Canyons (Chapter 4, Trip 2). One of the most popular spots for mountain biking in Orange County. Not all trails are open to bikes.

Emerald Canyon (Chapter 4, Trip 5). Ridgeline views plus an intimate canyon setting—this ride or run has it all.

Gilman Peak (Chapter 6, Trip 2). A short but challenging ascent on a graded roadway. Excellent views at the top.

Telegraph Canyon Traverse (Chapter 6, Trip 8). Moderate grades. Remarkably unspoiled, yet close to the city's edge.

Whiting Ranch Loop (Chapter 8, Trip 2). Moderate grades on mostly wide trails. A classic among mountain bikers.

North Main Divide Traverse (Chapter 12, Trip 4). Challenging trip up and over the northern crest of the Main Divide. Delightful views.

Harding Road (Chapter 12, Trips 7 & 8). Long climb to the Main Divide just north of Old Saddleback. Return the same way or continue along the Main Divide.

Indian Truck Trail (Chapter 12, Trip 13). The most scenic ascent by road to the Main Divide from the east.

San Juan Trail (Chapter 13, Trip 4). Ascend or descend 11 miles on a winding single-track trail.

Appendix 2
Urban and Regional Trails

Despite its automobile-dominated milieu, Orange County has made significant strides in the development of alternative transportation systems.

Cyclists and hikers, for example, can explore many miles of paved pathways along Orange County's oceanfront and rivers. The trails often follow nearly flat levees, and allow fairly pleasant travel through some of the county's more densely populated areas. The river paths include the Santa Ana River bike path all the way across the county into Riverside County, the San Diego Creek trail in Irvine, and the San Juan Creek trail in San Juan Capistrano. The El Cajon bike path in Yorba Linda traces the course of the former Anaheim Union Canal.

Orange County's general plan has long recognized the importance of setting aside parcels of land for parks, greenbelts, and trail corridors. This has proven quite feasible in the county's eastern and southern regions. County policy, in fact, requires that developers of large-scale projects dedicate substantial parcels of land for recreational and wildlife-protection purposes in exchange for the right to build. The Irvine Company, the single largest private owner of such lands, has created an entity called the Irvine Ranch Land Reserve, consisting of a 50,000-acre patchwork of existing and future park lands stretching across the county. Trails in the reserve's Upper Newport Bay, San Joaquin Wildlife Sanctuary, Crystal Cove State Park, Laguna Coast Wilderness Park, Irvine Regional Park, and Peters Canyon Regional Park areas have been described in this book. Other areas, such as Bommer Canyon, Limestone Canyon, Fremont Canyon, and Anaheim Canyon, are now open to the hiking, cycling, and equestrian public by means of guided tours given by The Nature Conservancy, which is serving as the reserve's administrative steward. Log on to www.irvineranchlandreserve.com for access and contact information.

A key component in developing regional trails is the establishment of linkages between the road and trail systems of Cleveland National Forest (Santa Ana Mountains) and the trail systems of both Orange and Riverside counties. This is an ongoing challenge, and it is sometimes frustrated (especially on the Riverside County side) by new subdivisions that have blocked access to routes up into the Santa Anas.

Since the trips in this book were selected primarily on the basis of being "afield," or away from populated areas, as well as being suitable for travel "afoot," I did not highlight quite a number of worthy trails in Orange County's urban areas and suburbs. You can find many of those with the help of Orange County Transportation Authority's free Orange County Bikeways Map, which is widely available at the county's regional and wilderness park offices. The map offers a comprehensive look at long-distance bikeways and multiuse trails, as well as striped or signed bike routes on road and street shoulders.

Another good, global source of information about Orange County's regional parks and trails is the County of Orange Harbors, Beaches, and Parks division's website: www.ocparks.com.

Appendix 3
Recommended Reading

Bailey, H.P., *The Climate of Southern California*, University of California Press, 1966. (Out of print)

Bakker, Elna, *An Island Called California*, 2nd edition, University of California Press, 1984.

Belzer, Thomas J., *Roadside Plants of Southern California*, Mountain Press Publishing Co., 1984.

California Coastal Commission, *California Coastal Access Guide*, 6th edition, University of California Press, 2003.

California Division of Mines and Geology, *Geologic Map of California—Santa Ana Sheet*, 1965.

National Geographic Society, *Field Guide to the Birds of North America*, 4th edition, 2002.

Peterson, P. Victor, *Native Trees of Southern California*, University of California Press, 1972.

Raven, Peter H., *Native Shrubs of Southern California*, University of California Press, 1976.

Rundel, Phillip W., and John R. Gustafson, *Introduction to the Plant Life of Southern California: Coast to Foothills*, University of California Press, 2005.

Schad, Jerry, *Afoot and Afield in Los Angeles County*, 2nd edition, Wilderness Press, 2000.

——, *Afoot and Afield in San Diego County*, 3rd edition, Wilderness Press, 1998.

Schoenherr, Allan A., *A Natural History of California*, Univeristy of California Press, 1995.

Sharp, Robert P., *Coastal Southern California* (geology guide), Kendall/ Hunt Publishing Company, 1978.

Sharp, Robert P., *Geology Field Guide to Southern California*, William C. Brown Co., 1972.

Stephenson, Terry E., *Shadows of Old Saddleback: Tales of the Santa Ana Mountains*, (reprint of 1931 edition), Rasmussen Press, 1974.

Appendix 4
Local Organizations

Sea and Sage Audubon Society
P.O. Box 5477
Irvine, CA 92616
(949) 261-7963
(Sponsors field trips and bird walks in Orange County's coastal wetlands and foothill canyons. Maintains an office at the San Joaquin Wildlife Sanctuary.)

Sierra Club Orange County Group
P.O. Box 6647
Orange, CA 92867
(949) 631-3140
(Sponsors day hikes and camping trips throughout Orange County; advocates preservation of open spaces; plans and maintains trails in the Trabuco District of Cleveland National Forest.)

Amigos de Bolsa Chica
16531 Bolsa Chica St. Suite 312
Huntington Beach, CA 92649
(714) 840-1575
(Activities associated with Bolsa Chica Ecological Reserve.)

Crystal Cove Interpretive Association
P.O. Box 4352
Laguna Beach, CA 92652
(949) 497-7648
(Activities associated with Crystal Cove State Park.)

Hills for Everyone
P.O. Box 9835
Brea, CA 92822
(714) 687-1555
(Advocates land acquisition for wildlife habitat and recreation in the Chino and Puente hills area.)

Chino Hills State Park Interpretive Association
4195 Chino Hills Parkway, Suite E-454
Chino Hills, CA 91709
(951) 780-6222
(Activities associated with Chino Hills State Park.)

The Nature Conservancy of California
1400 Quail St., Suite 130
Newport Beach, CA 92660
(949) 263-0933
(Manages and sponsors guided hikes on Nature Conservancy and Irvine Company open-space reserves.)

Appendix 5
Information Sources

Parks, Preserves, and Agencies

Aliso and Wood Canyons Wilderness Park (**AWCWP**) . . . .(949) 923-2200

Bolsa Chica Ecological Reserve (**BCER**) . . . .(714) 846-1114

Carbon Canyon Regional Park (**CCRP**) . . . .(714) 973-3160

Caspers Wilderness Park (**CWP**) . . . .(949) 923-2210

Crystal Cove State Park (**CCSP**) . . . .(949) 494-3539

Chino Hills State Park (**CHSP**). . . . .(951) 780-6222

Cleveland National Forest
   Trabuco Ranger District (**CNF/TD**) . . . .(951) 736-1811
   1147 E. Sixth Street
   Corona, CA 92879

Cleveland National Forest
   El Cariso Visitor Information Office . . . .(951) 678-3700
   32353 Ortega Highway
   Lake Elsinore, CA 92330

Irvine Regional Park (**IRP**) . . . .(714) 973-6835

Laguna Coast Wilderness Park (**LCWP**) . . . .(949) 923-2235

Oak Canyon Nature Center (**OCNC**) . . . .(714) 998-8380

Ocean Institute, Dana Point (**OIDP**) . . . .(949) 496-2274

O'Neill Regional Park (**ONRP**) . . . .(949) 923-2260

Peters Canyon Regional Park (**PCRP**) . . . .(714) 973-6611

Riley Wilderness Park (**RWP**) . . . .(949) 923-2265

San Clemente State Beach (**SCSB**) . . . .(949) 492-3156

San Joaquin Wildlife Sanctuary (**SJWS**) . . . .(949) 261-7963

San Onofre State Beach (**SOSB**) . . . .(949) 492-4872

Santa Rosa Plateau Ecological Reserve (**SRPER**) . . . .(951) 677-6951

Santiago Oaks Regional Park (**SORP**) . . . .(714) 973-6620

Talbert Nature Preserve (**TNP**) . . . .(949) 923-2250

The Nature Conservancy (**TNC**) . . . .(949) 263-0933

Upper Newport Bay Ecological Reserve (**UNBER**) . . . .(949) 923-2290

Whiting Ranch Wilderness Park (**WRWP**) . . . .(949) 923-2245

Map Sources

Adventure 16 Wilderness Outfitters . . . .(714) 427-0410
2937 Bristol St.
Costa Mesa, CA 92626

Allied Map Services . . . .(714) 532-4300
966 North Main
Orange, CA 92867

Cleveland National Forest—see previous section

Recreational Equipment, Inc. (REI) . . . .(714) 543-4142
1411 Village Way
(McFadden Place)
Santa Ana, CA 92705

Index

About the Author

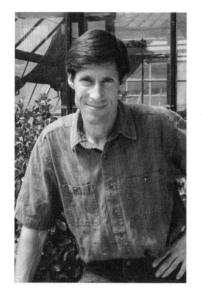

Jerry Schad's several parallel careers have encompassed interests ranging from astronomy and teaching to photography and writing. He teaches astronomy and physical science at San Diego Mesa College, and currently chairs the Physical Sciences Department there.

Schad has run or hiked many thousands of miles of distinct trails throughout California, in the Southwest, and in Mexico. He is a sub-24-hour finisher of Northern California's 100-mile Western States Endurance Run, and has served in a leadership capacity for outdoor excursions as close as San Diego County and as far away as Madagascar. More information can be found at Schad's website: www.skyphoto.com.

BOOKS BY JERRY SCHAD

50 Southern California Bicycle Trips
101 Hikes in Southern California
Adventure Running
Afoot & Afield in Los Angeles County
Afoot & Afield in Orange County
Afoot & Afield in San Diego County
Back Roads and Hiking Trails, The Santa Cruz Mountains
Backcountry Roads and Trails, San Diego County
California Deserts
Cycling Orange County
Cycling San Diego
Physical Science: A Unified Approach
Top Trails Los Angeles
Trail Runner's Guide San Diego

Other Jerry Schad Books from Wilderness Press

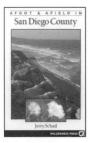

Afoot & Afield in San Diego County

San Diego's best-selling comprehensive hiking guidebook, featuring 220 detailed descriptions of every trail worth taking, from Torrey Pines to the Carrizo Badlands and beyond. Catalogs the best trips along the coast, through the foothills, up the mountains, and across the desert.

ISBN 0-89997-229-2

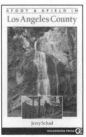

Afoot & Afield in Los Angeles County

Covering all the best L.A. adventures, from strolling along at Malibu Lagoon State Beach to trekking up a mountain on Catalina Island. Close to 200 trips explore the City of Angels' own backyard, traveling through a variety of climate zones and revealing a remarkably diverse array of plant and animal life.

ISBN 0-89997-267-5

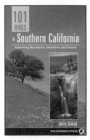

101 Hikes in Southern California

The book that proves there's more to SoCal than theme parks and strip malls. From the San Gabriel Mountains to the Anza-Borrego Desert and everywhere in between, this guide offers an incredible selection of exciting trips covering scores of hidden places just beyond the urban horizon.

ISBN 0-89997-351-5

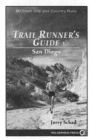

Trail Runner's Guide San Diego

A comprehensive guide to running the myriad trails of sun-soaked San Diego, from the beach at La Jolla to the summit of Palomar Mountain. Runners and hikers alike will appreciate the detailed descriptions of 50 exhilarating routes. Includes climate and topography tips, maps, photos, and more.

ISBN 0-89997-308-6

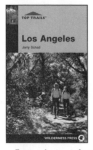

Top Trails: Los Angeles

Highly visual guide to 48 of the Southland's best trails in the greater LA metro area, from Malibu to the Hollywood Hills, San Jacinto Peak to the San Fernando Valley. Includes trail feature tables, don't-get-lost milestones, maps for every trip, and more.

ISBN 0-89997-347-7

For ordering information, contact your local bookseller or Wilderness Press, www.wildernesspress.com